SHIPWRECKS OF THE WIGHT

by

J.C. Medland

This book is dedicated to all those who have risked their lives to save those in peril on the sea.

Printed and Published by West Island Printers Ltd., Afton Road, Freshwater, Isle of Wight.©1986

ISBN 0 9511498 0 6

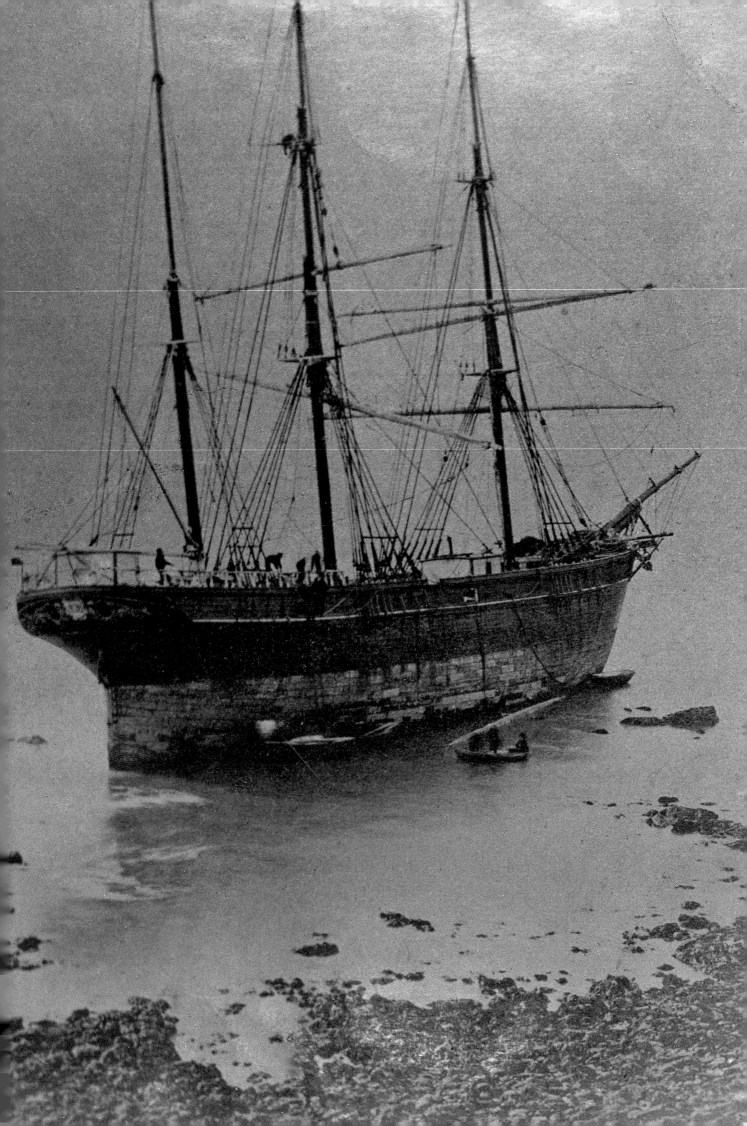

Contents

(Facing page) The Catalina stranded in Binnel Bay, 1878. (Courtesy of Viv Spencer).

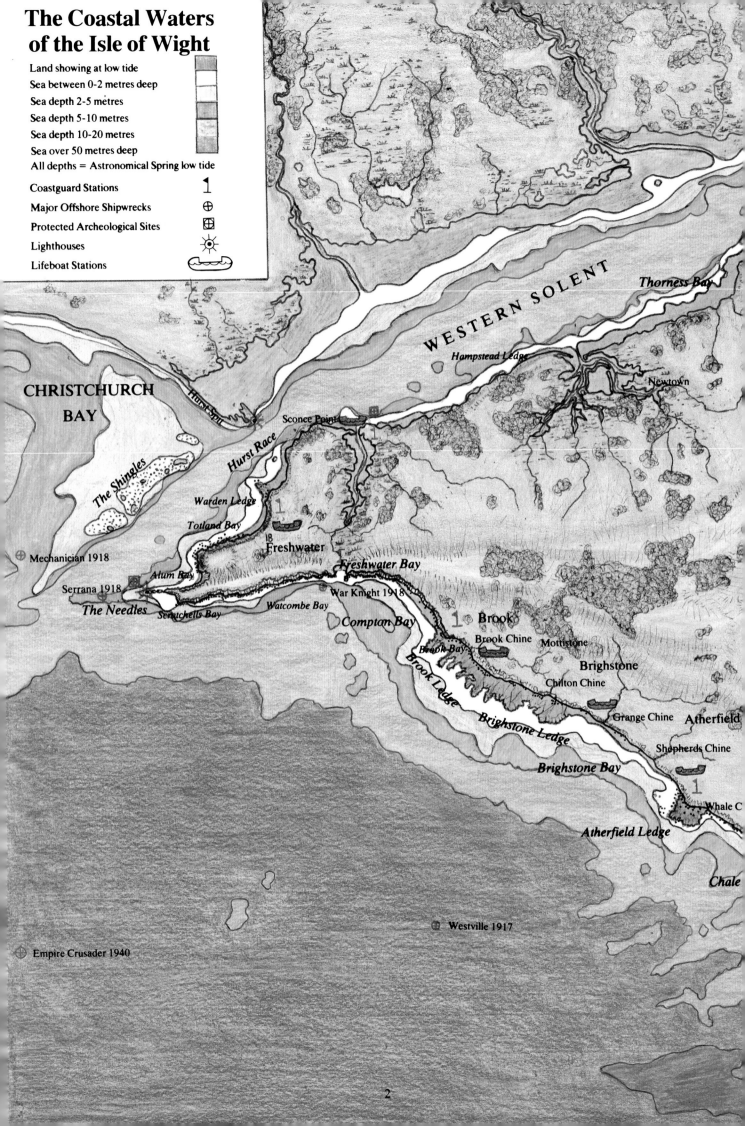

The Coastal Waters of the Isle of Wight

Land showing at low tide
Sea between 0-2 metres deep
Sea depth 2-5 metres
Sea depth 5-10 metres
Sea depth 10-20 metres
Sea over 50 metres deep
All depths = Astronomical Spring low tide

Coastguard Stations
Major Offshore Shipwrecks
Protected Archeological Sites
Lighthouses
Lifeboat Stations

CHRISTCHURCH BAY

WESTERN SOLENT

Thorness Bay

Hampstead Ledge

Newtown

Hurst Spit

Sconce Point

Hurst Race

The Shingles

Warden Ledge

Totland Bay

Freshwater

Mechanician 1918

Alum Bay

Freshwater Bay

Serrana 1918

The Needles

Scratchells Bay

Watcombe Bay

War Knight 1918

Brook

Brook Chine

Mottistone

Compton Bay

Brook Bay

Brighstone

Chilton Chine

Brook Ledge

Brighstone Ledge

Grange Chine

Atherfield

Shepherds Chine

Brighstone Bay

Whale C

Atherfield Ledge

Chale

Westville 1917

Empire Crusader 1940

2

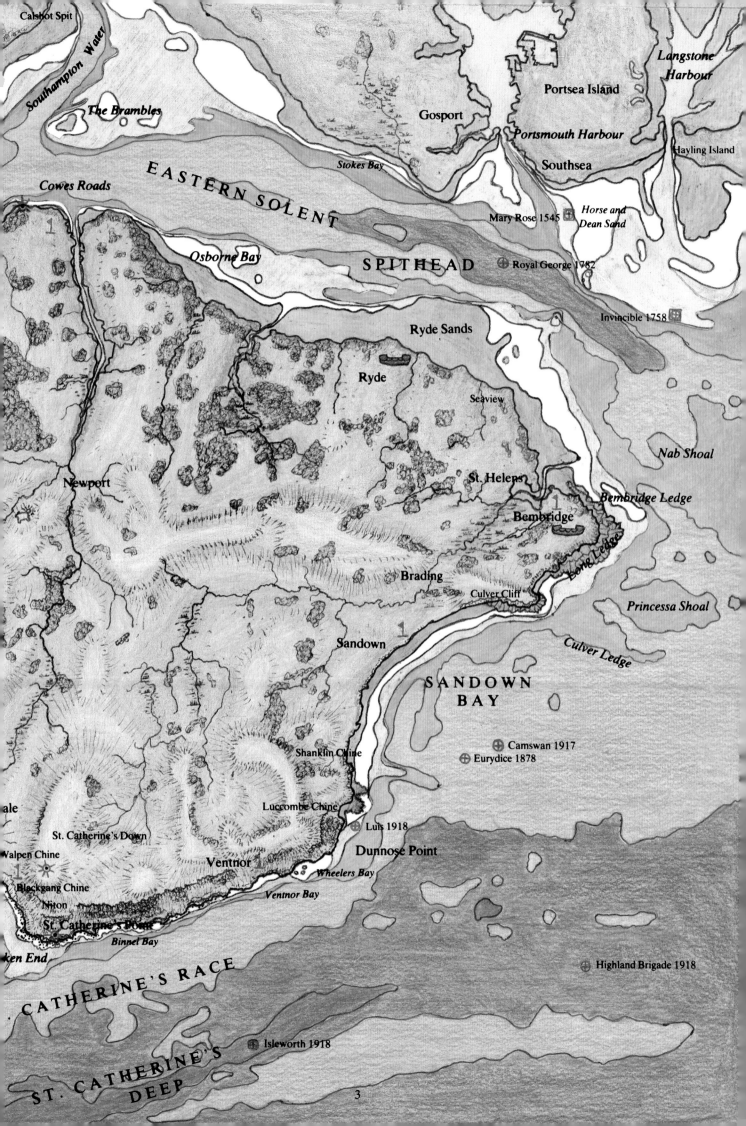

Calshot Spit

Southampton Water

The Brambles

EASTERN SOLENT

Cowes Roads

Osborne Bay

SPITHEAD

Stokes Bay

Portsea Island

Gosport

Portsmouth Harbour

Southsea

Langstone Harbour

Hayling Island

Mary Rose 1545

Horse and Dean Sand

Royal George 1782

Invincible 1758

Ryde Sands

Ryde

Seaview

Nab Shoal

Newport

St. Helens

Bembridge

Bembridge Ledge

Long Ledge

Brading

Princessa Shoal

Culver Cliff

Culver Ledge

Sandown

SANDOWN BAY

Camswan 1917

Eurydice 1878

Shanklin Chine

Luccombe Chine

Luis 1918

St. Catherine's Down

Dunnose Point

ale

Walpen Chine

Ventnor

Wheelers Bay

Blackgang Chine

Ventnor Bay

Niton

St. Catherine's Point

Highland Brigade 1918

Binnel Bay

ken End

CATHERINE'S RACE

Isleworth 1918

ST. CATHERINE'S DEEP

3

Guide to Sail

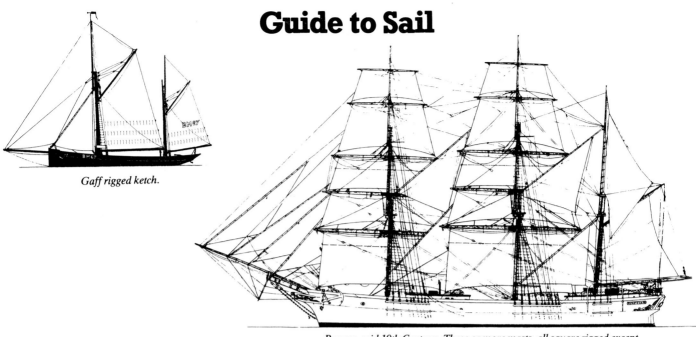

Gaff rigged ketch.

Barque, mid 19th Century. Three or more masts, all square rigged except the mizzen mast which is rigged fore and aft.

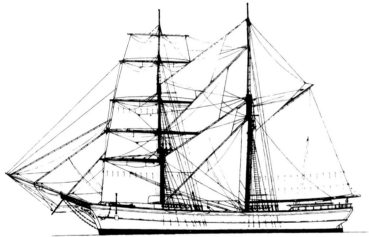

A squaresail schooner. There were many types of schooner, usually two masted and fore and aft rigged. Foremast shorter than mizzen.

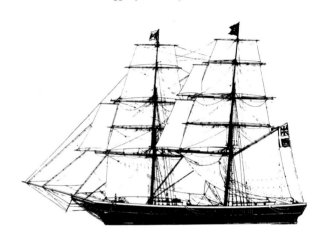

Brig: Two masted and square rigged with gaff mainsail. Mid 19th Century.

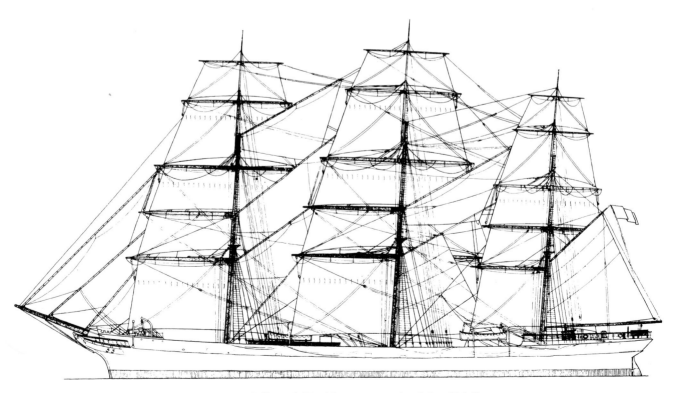

Full rigged ship. All masts square rigged. Late 19th Century.

Introduction

For around four thousand years the Isle of Wight has witnessed the destruction of untold thousands of vessels along its shores, and the deaths of hundreds of mariners. The sheer volume of shipwrecks is staggering. The Admiralty has found 4,000 wrecks in the area covered by the chart 'Solent Approaches.' Many more have not yet been discovered, (including huge ships like the 9,044 ton *S.S. Mechanician,* which was lost in 1917 and disappeared into a shoal of shingle). These offshore wrecks, vessels which foundered in storms or were sunk in war or by collision, are only a fraction of the far greater number stranded and wrecked on the Island itself. Most of these escaped, sometimes on the next high tide or by jettisoning their cargo, or through a tow, but many others were driven further inshore, smashed on the rocks and strewn along the shore.

The seas around the Island have been busy with shipping for well over 2,000 years. The English Channel has long been a highway for traders ferrying goods along the coast, to the continent, and in the last 500 years to the four corners of the Earth. Since Roman times warships have used the splendid harbour of Portsmouth and the Spithead anchorage, perfectly strategically placed to dominate the Channel. The Island itself has been a natural base for generations of fishing boats, ferries, pilot vessels and pleasure boats; and in more lawless times, pirate ships and smuggling boats.

The Island's 60 mile coastline is unevenly scattered with a succession of appalling marine hazards which leave little room for luck and good seamanship in adverse conditions. The long Solent shoreline from Seaview to Yarmouth is the safest stretch with its gentle shoreline and fine harbours, sheltered from the prevailing winds by the Island's long ridge of high chalk downs. The only hazards are the tidal currents and sudden squalls that can whip the placid Solent into a raging tempest like that which capsized the Ryde lifeboat *Selina* in 1907.

The Solent and Southampton Water are drowned river valleys. The mouth of the old River Solent became the Spithead, for centuries the anchorage from which the Royal Navy sailed to dominate the three oceans of the world. Despite being in the sheltered lee of the Island the Spithead has seen two of the greatest tragedies in maritime history, the loss of the flagships *Mary Rose* and *Royal George,* both of which capsized through mismanagement with the loss of about 1,500 people in all.

The Perils of the Western Wight

At the other end of the Solent danger is posed by the fast tidal current, especially west of Yarmouth. The tide enters the Solent from both ends, but it mostly escapes through the narrow western channel, only a mile wide at Hurst Spit. The racing current achieves a speed of five knots and reaches the sea through a succession of races (the open sea version of rapids) off Sconce Point, Hurst Spit and the Needles. Once past Hurst the sea cannot disperse into Christchurch Bay but is held tight against the shore by The Shingles, a mountainous shoal of pebbles three miles long and almost as high as the sea. At high tide small craft can sail right over it but otherwise it is a dangerous feature, constantly moving and threatening to trap the unwary. At the time of writing the 1,000 ton *Tutonia* spent several tides grounded there before she was hauled off. Most ships grounded there in the past escaped with the tide but if caught by a rising swell any vessel was in great danger. Many people have perished on this broad wilderness of pebbles.

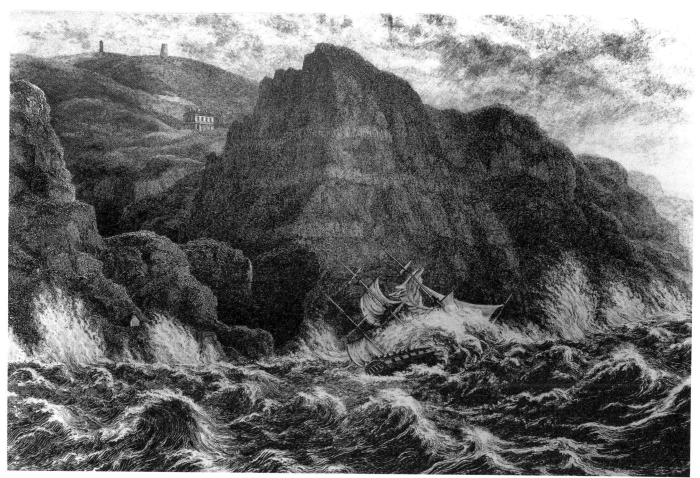

The full rigged West Indiaman Clarendon, wrecked at Blackgang Chine in 1836. She was completely destroyed by just four seas and all but three of the 26 people aboard were killed.

Until the last century the Island's coast from Yarmouth to the Needles was an unbroken stretch of high overgrown cliffs and boulder strewn beaches. Warden Ledge sticks out into the main channel for about half a mile midway along the coast. Beyond the three jagged chalk stacks of the Needles lies the Needles Bridge, a ridge of chalk that Lord Mottistone once called "the terror of all mariners."

The Back of the Wight

Between the Needles and St. Catherine's Point lies the most treacherous stretch of the Island's shore, as the long sweep of the Back of the Wight forms a bay 18 miles long into which countless numbers of vessels have been embayed (trapped by the wind). This coast is notorious for blinding fogs, a steady ocean swell and driving south-westerly storms from the Atlantic Ocean. If one sailed straight out to sea from here the next landfall would be Brazil, 3,000 miles away, making this the most exposed of all the Island's coasts.

This whole shoreline offers no consolation to the storm pressed mariner. There is no shelter, only the false harbour of Freshwater Bay where many vessels have sought safety only to be torn apart on the shallow chalk bar which runs beneath the mouth of the bay.

The towering chalk cliffs, which average 300 feet high and stretch for five miles from Alum Bay to Compton, offer little solace to the shipwrecked mariner. They are succeeded by deeply eroded sandstone cliffs which run from Compton to Chale with only two points of easy access to the beach, at Brook Chine and nearby Grange Chine at Brighstone. From Grange Chine onwards there is no point of easy access to the shore until one reaches Ventnor, 13 miles distant. In Compton Bay the steep chalk beach is succeeded by long slimey fingers of clay and smooth rock slabs that extend up to half a mile out at low tide and continue for six miles to Brighstone Bay, being known as Brook and Brighstone Ledges. These ugly and treacherous features have claimed countless ships and lives.

About two miles further along the steep shelving shore from Brighstone Ledge lie the even more treacherous rocks of "the dreaded Atherfield Ledge." Although only half a mile square, the ledge occupies a deadly position, protruding into the powerful south-easterly coastal current. As it lies in the middle of the great western bay it becomes the focal point for the incoming tide. An extraordinary number of vessels have found themselves grounded here, and very few have escaped. The place is like a ship's graveyard, still littered with the corroded remains of its victims. The reason for this grisly record is the uneven nature of the ledges surface, a complex shambles of rock slabs, ridges, scattered boulders and sharp reefs. The incoming sea becomes a frenzied chaos of terrifying breakers when the wind rises. This has been the scene of many tragic wrecks and extraordinary rescues.

On past Atherfield one comes to Chale Bay. "The Receiver General of Wrecks for the Isle of Wight" as 'The Times' once called it. James Wheeler's log of the Eighteenth Century and Fred Mew's book 'Back of the Wight' give us some idea of the sheer volume of wrecks along this forbidding shore. There are only four points of access to the interior, two steep gashes cut into the cliff face by streams, Whale and Walpen Chines, the deeply eroded Ladder Chine and the highest and greatest of them all, Blackgang Chine, once home of a gang of cut-throat smugglers.

Rocken End to Bembridge Ledge

At the southern end of Chale Bay the land suddenly rears up some 500 feet in a series of deeply eroded and terraced iron tinted cliffs that culminate in the boulder strewn chaos of Rocken End where the currents are faster, the beach slopes steeper, and there is faint hope of any assistance from the shore.

If the embayed mariner manages to avoid the gnarled outcrops of Rocken End he is sometimes faced with an even more horrifying danger, St. Catherine's Race, one of the worst around the British Isles. It is caused by the eastward moving sea being forced between the bulk of the Island's southern coast and a long parallel ridge three miles offshore and rising to just 15 metres below the surface. Between the two the sea has scoured a narrow channel of extraordinary depth, St. Catherine's Deep. South and west of Rocken End lie massive chasms up to 300 feet deep which add to the

turbulance and account for the extraordinary behaviour of the sea hereabouts. In certain conditions mountainous seas erupt from the depths and charge each other at right angles. Ships swamped and sunk in the race often disappeared with all hands and without any trace of wreckage.

There is no shelter for the storm bound mariner all along the southern coast which rears up steep and overgrown like some tropical volcanic island. The Undercliff is still largely wilderness and the exposed bays are littered with boulders and offer no hope. Attempts to build harbours at Puckaster Cove and Ventnor Bay in Victorian times both failed due to the ferocity of the weather.

The east coast of the southern Wight is again steep and treacherous with high cliffs. There is limited access to the beach at Luccombe Chine. Past Horse Ledge lies the wide peaceful expanse of Sandown Bay. This is sheltered from the prevailing south-westerlies but is fully exposed to terrible continental storms that sometimes sweep across the Channel with hurricane force winds. Most vessels driven ashore on the sandy beach can be easily salvaged but there have been many total wrecks and courageous rescues along this gentle looking stretch of coastline.

The eastern Wight also has its share of dangers, the 300 foot Culver Cliff, the broad rock shelf of Long Ledge, and offshore shoals and rocks. The most dangerous is the fearful submerged ridge of Bembridge Ledge, lying just offshore, and another renowned killer.

Longshoremen to Lifeboatmen

These days shipwrecks are rare events. One modern freighter has the capacity of a score of old merchant ships, drastically reducing the number of vessels engaged in trade. Accidents are rarer thanks to the sophisticated navigation equipment operated on board ships and by Trinity House and the Coastguard, and ships are built stronger and equipped with powerful engines to prevent them becoming total wrecks. However, it is only in the last 70 years that the Island's marine hazards have been tamed.

For centuries shipwreck was a major source of income for the longshoremen of the Island's rugged coasts. Longshoremen were a tough breed who made their living by fishing, a little farm labouring, and in taking every opportunity that the sea could offer to enrich their subsistence lifestyle, becoming pirates, smugglers, and salvors. There is a well known local legend which claimed that some longshoremen deliberately enticed ships onto the rocks to murder their crews and steal their cargoes. Thankfully there is no historical evidence to support this myth, except perhaps in the Thirteenth Century when the murder of shipwrecked crews was sometimes practised.

This legend tends to obscure the fact that these longshoremen were responsible for the saving of thousands of people who would have otherwise perished on the Island's cruel coasts. Some of them sacrificed their lives for these people who they had never met nor seen before. In the Nineteenth Century state institutions like the Coastguard and Trinity House, became increasingly concerned with preventing wrecks. Moreover, the Royal National Lifeboat Institution, a national charity manned by volunteer crews taken from the families of the longshoremen, took the brunt of the rescue work.

The R.N.L.I. has a glorious record of success on the Island saving 1,827 lives in 126 years, largely thanks to the perennial support of the Island's people as volunteers and donors. The R.N.L.I. needs to receive around £23,000,000 every year to continue its outstanding work. Every penny helps.

What follows is not a concise and comprehensive history of shipwrecks around the Island, but rather an attempt to illustrate the general subject, highlight some particular wrecks, and recall some of the instances of selfless courage, self-sacrifice and heroism that otherwise might be forgotten.

The Waters of the Wight to 1066

It was not until the end of the last Ice Age that the sea level rose to drown the valleys of the River Solent and its tributaries, the Test, Itchen, Medina and the Eastern and Western Yars. Nevertheless, the Wight remained connected along the chalk ridge which ran from the Needles to Hengistbury Head, near Christchurch. The flooded river valleys provided some of the finest harbours in the world and the sheltered waters of the Solent made it a perfect place for shipbuilding, sailing and trade.

Around 1,500 B.C. British tribes were trading goods from Scandinavia to Spain. (By this time the Island, then called Yns Yr Wyth, was fully separated from the mainland). Some mariners even came from the Mediterranean to trade for British metals, especially tin.

In the centuries approaching the time of Christ the Island assumed a central position in the growing cross-Channel trade. Two commercial networks developed, one between the Regnum people of Sussex, and Flanders; and one between the Durotriges of Dorset, and Brittany and Normandy. The Dorotriges main port was nearby Hengistbury Head where British metals, slaves and hides were exchanged for fine Mediterranean pottery, ornaments, arms and coins. The two British tribes had their own coinage, leaving the Island perfectly placed as a point of interchange between the two.

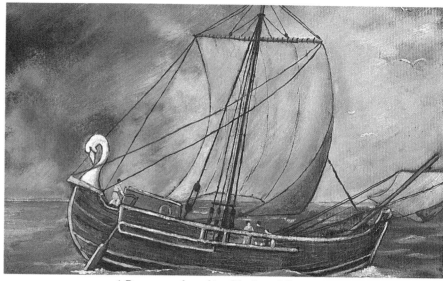

A Roman merchant ship of the Second Century AD.

Ancient Wreck at Yarmouth?

A few years ago some Yarmouth fishermen discovered fragments of Roman pottery in their nets just east of Yarmouth Pier. Archaelogists have been painstakingly working the site ever since and have brought to the surface about 60 fragments of pottery and tile, mostly from broken amphorae, ancient storage vessels much used in Mediterranean maritime commerce. Few conclusions can be drawn at this stage but the artefacts, which come from all over the Roman world, have been dated from the First Century B.C., a hundred years before the Roman conquest.

It is possible that these fragments come from a pre-Roman shipwreck but no trace of one has been found and it is most unlikely that any pieces of it would remain after two millenia in the strong tidal current. If it was a pre-Roman wreck we have some idea of what it would have been like thanks to a description written by Julius Ceasar when he conquered France and attacked Britain in 55 B.C. He described the ships of the Channel as built of thick oak planks and powered entirely by sail, "Their bulk rendered them safe against ramming while their height placed them beyond the reach of our missiles and grappling irons . . . they were not only more seaworthy but could heave-to in shallow water."

The Passing of Rome

A century later the Romans invaded and conquered Britain which developed into one of the wealthiest provinces of the western empire. Many villas were established on the Island which exported grain in return for the luxury goods of the empire. The New Forest became an important area for the production of fine red pottery and the seas around the Island must have been busy with local and Roman shipping for the first three hundred years of imperial rule. Many of these vessels must have perished on the wild and rugged shores of the Island, one at least was wrecked on the Needles. In 1982 divers excavating a site at Goose Rock discovered a number of Roman coins there.

By the Fourth Century the Empire was breaking up. The economy collapsed and the state was unable to prevent devastating attacks by German pirates and raiders. The Imperial Channel Fleet repeatedly mutinied and the army pulled out leaving the Britons to the invading German tribes. The Dark Ages saw a collapse of trade. The only shipwrecks would have been the slim fearful longships of the Germanic and Norse peoples who devastated the Channel coasts in a series of raids and migratory invasions. The last Viking attack on the Island was driven off by King Harold in 1066. By then the English had a considerable fleet, but Harold was obliged to disband it shortly before William sailed from Normandy to take the English crown at the Battle of Hastings.

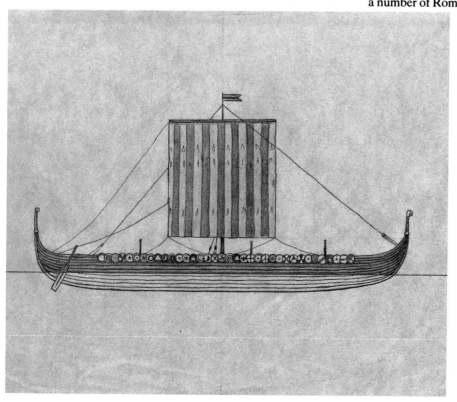

A small Viking longship of the Ninth Century.

Wrecks of the Medieval Wight

In the centuries following the Norman Conquest western Europe enjoyed a period of relative peace. The migrations and invasions of nomad peoples subsided. Population and wealth slowly grew, and given the increased security provided by the authority of the Catholic Church and the growing power of the Crown, trade began to develop. Large scale textile manufacturing developed in Flanders and Italy, and with it a voracious demand for English wool. By the 14th century England exported 8,000,000 fleeces every year, much of it through Southampton, which became England's second port after London. The wool of Dorset, Somerset and Devon was shipped to Southampton through the Needles Channel. That of Gloucestershire, Berkshire and Wiltshire came by barge down the Itchen from Winchester. In Southampton Water they tied up alongside the ships of the French and Spanish convoys, and exchanged their cargoes of English wool for wine. The Venetian oared galley fleet also visited Southampton every year until 1536.

There was also lively local trade. Yarmouth, Shalfleet, Newtown, Newport, Wootton and Brading all grew to importance, at this time when ships were small, round shallow 'cogs' of not more than 100 tons.

Many of these ships must have perished on the shores of the Medieval Wight. Ship design was primitive, little refined from the long ships of the Dark Ages. Navigation was still a matter of hugging the coastline and dodging the reefs. Many were embayed and wrecked on the Island as we can see by the complex arrangements made to share out the proceeds. 'Wreck' was a major source of income. Every parish was distorted to give it a slice of shoreline, and a share in the spoils. Leases and title deeds specified the right of the owner to a proportion of the salvage. The Lords of the Island took the rest.

Island Wreckers

The people of the Island were very poor. They lived on the wild western fringe of Christian civilisation scattered in mud and thatch hamlets around the ragged shores of a densely forested land. Even the lifestyle of the Lords in the cold, stone castle of Carisbrooke would strike us as deprived. Reliant on fickle weather, exposed to terrible attacks from bloodthirsty pirates, they scraped a mean living from fishing and the land, supplemented by trade and salvage. Shipwrecks were a Godsend to these people, bringing ashore wealth and merchandise beyond their dreams. There were no records kept before the 13th century. Mariners crawling from the surf were often clubbed to death so that their cargoes could be seized with no questions asked.

In 1224 this activity came to the attention of the Bishop of Winchester. He was enraged and ordered the clergy to preach three times a year against those who "prevented the shipwrecked from saving their own lives." This is the closest we come to the Island legend of deliberate wrecking. Professional wreckers would light fires to attract ships onto the rocks. Such men certainly existed in the Hebrides, on the Cornish coasts and the west coast of Ireland, as late as the 17th century but there is no evidence of this on the Island. However, given the moral standards of the times, it is hardly out of the question.

As time went by the Crown was forced to take an interest in the growing trade of wreck-theft that had become established on the Island. The merchants who provided Medieval kings with cash loans, demanded protection. In 1231 Henry III set up an enquiry on behalf of Osbert Percehays. One of his ships had been driven by a storm to beach itself near Freshwater. She was not a real wreck, but a crowd of men came down the cliff and stole the whole cargo of Lampreys (eel like fish, a great delicacy of the time).

In 1293 Isabella de Fortibus, last of the feudal overlords of the Island, died without heirs and the Island reverted to the Crown, as did the rights of salvage. It is from this time that we have some records that concern large ships which reached posterity through the courts of the Crown or the church.

In 1301 the King and the local landlords split the proceeds from the remains of a ship from Calais, 'broken on the rocks' at Compton. There was not a lot of it left, selling for the grand sum of 47 shillings, a penny and a farthing.

The First Lighthouse

In 1313 occurred the most famous of the Island's Medieval wrecks, the *St. Mary of Bayonne*. The Ship of the Blessed Mary was sailing from Bayonne in Gascony with a cargo of 147 barrels of white wine from the Duchy of Aquitaine. She was bound for Picardy, where the wine would be delivered to the monastry of Livers. However, the *Mary* was blown off course, far to the north, and on April 22nd she was driven ashore in Chale Bay, in the remote and wild wastes of the 'Back of the Wight.'

The crew managed to get the bulk of the cargo ashore, and naturally they had plenty of help in this from the villagers of 'Cheal' who ran down the chines to grab or buy what they could. The best organised of these happy scavengers was Walter de Godeton, Lord of Chale, who descended to the chaotic scene of drunken robbery with his retainers and bought 53 barrels from the crew, who were probably petrified and would have given them away. When the ship's owners were informed they were not pleased. As Gascons

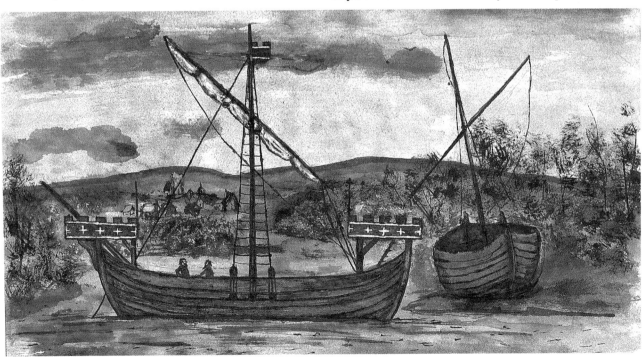

A medieval ship, converted for war by building 'castles' fore and aft.

8

they were also subjects of the English King, Edward II, and they demanded justice. Edward acted promptly. The courts of Southampton summoned Godeton and three others to its sessions. With a reply that was to become characteristic of Islanders facing charges they said that they were not there, and refused three summonses. Finally they arrived at Winchester and were heavily fined. Walter had to raise a huge sum of over 267 marks, with 20 marks damages, something like £9,000 in modern terms. Walter must have been a rich man as his fines were paid by June 24th, 1314. It seemed that the matter was then done with, but unfortunately for Walter his misdemeanour had come to the attention of Pope Clement V, God's spokesman on Earth, then believed to hold the keys of Heaven and Hell.

Sacrilege!

Godeton was accused of 'sacrilege.' He had to be punished. He was lucky to avoid excommunication. Instead the church courts sentenced him to a penance. He was ordered to build a lighthouse on the 'Montem de Cheal' and with it a chantry where a priest would live and sing prayers for the soul of Walter, and his family, and for those lost at sea. He had to set aside rents to keep it running in perpetuity.

Walter fulfilled all the conditions. On the bleak high hill that rears up sharply from the flat lands of Chale, a hermitage was already established. Here Walter built the tower, thirty-five and a half feet high, octangular without and quadrangular within, with a pyramidal roof. It is the second oldest surviving lighthouse in Britain. It was completed in 1328 and dedicated to St. Catherine. Next to it once stood the austere chapel where generations of priests prayed and collected faggots for the beacon which was kept burning for 212 years.

Thinking of these early public servants Fred Mew wrote, "On this desolate and windswept spot, far from other habitations, and usually shrouded in dense fog one marvels at the piety of these priests and monks who kept watch and ward there over the centuries, and the devotion which inspired them to do it." In the 1530's the lighthouse was closed due to the dissolution of the monastries. In the 18th century Richard Worsley added the buttresses to keep it from falling down.

One other reminder of these far off days is Gottens Farm, once Godeton Manor, Walter's home.

Wreck, Theft and Salvage

In 1320 another foreign ship, the *Saint Mary of Santander*, after being wrecked 'near Yarmouth' was set upon and her cargo seized. The owners pressed charges and 50 people were charged with 'the misuse of wrecked goods' including 'Henrye le parsonne of Mottestone.' Six men refused the summons to Southampton and were declared 'outlaws.' The offenders disappeared and the court found that they had no property which they could seize.

In 1324 the Plantagenet law of wrecks was finalised. It stated that if any man or beast escaped from a shipwreck alive, the owners could claim the salvaged goods if they applied within a year and a day. This was a poorly drawn up law. It proved to be an invitation to murder, so that a ship's goods could be legally stolen and it remained on the statute book for over three centuries.

In 1335 and 1336 two more large foreign wrecks were followed by organised robberies of the cargo. The *Ship of Jesus Christ* was raided by at least 45 men who came from as far afield as Christchurch and Portsmouth, showing that wrecks had become a regional industry, with a wide criminal network. Among the 45 accused was a de Godeton, possibly Walter's son.

In 1341 a Spanish ship foundered off a coast where salvage was reserved to the king. To the anger of the royal minions, armed men in boats rowed up and prodded the floating wine barrels out to sea where they could be claimed as flotsam by anyone.

In the latter half of the century the volume of trade declined thanks to the beginning of the 'Hundred Years War' against France. Edward III began by arresting every ship over a certain tonnage to add to his navy. He also licensed pirates to prey on French shipping. They did not distinguish too well between enemies and allies, nor did they observe truces. As a result the region sank into lawlessness and the great foreign ships stayed away. One victim of the times was the *Saint Marie Rose* which was sailing from Spain to England with a cargo of wine and honey when she was caught in a storm and driven to take shelter in the Solent. Master Gomez Peritz thought he was safe until his ship was

boarded and looted by pirates, who turned out to be the Crown's Stewards.

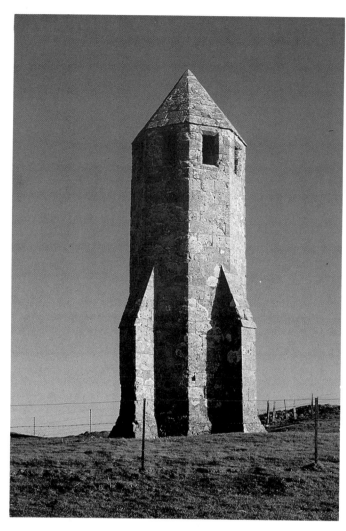

St. Catherine's Oratory, the Island's first known lighthouse; completed in 1328.

Another victim was the *Maudeleyn,* grounded off the Island in 1375 while en route from Flanders to Valencia, in Aragon, with 900 quarters of wheat. Grain was scarce as a French attack was expected so King Edward requisitioned the cargo and sold it in Southampton.

The war also affected the local carrying trade. Each side launched devastating cross-channel attacks. The five old villages of Freshwater and the main port and capital, Newtown, were obliterated by French raids, along with many other Island settlements.

As stable conditions returned in the next century the Spanish and Italian carracks began to return laden with wine, and we again have records of some of them being wrecked. A Breton ship loaded with claret was lost in October 1399. In 1409 a carrack from Saona, Italy, was beached near 'les Nedeles,' loaded with wine, oil and wax. Another carrack sank off the Island in 1447.

In 1463 *La Maudeleyn* came ashore with wine and a general cargo. The master felt secure as he had letters of safe conduct from King Edward IV. They did him little good. Pirates and thieves came aboard and stole the cargo and the letters.

As the 15th century progressed and the control of the Crown spread, the Island's pirates and wreck stealers faded into history. The Island became a more civilised place, run by gentlemen like the Worsleys and Oglanders. Unfortunately, with the criminals go all legal records of shipwrecks for the next two centuries. There is one exception: the *Mary Rose.*

The Mary Rose

On the evening of October 11th, 1982, the King's Ship *Mary Rose,* entered Portsmouth Harbour to the cheers of thousands of onlookers, after an absence of three months, and four hundred and thirty seven years. The story of this Tudor flagship is without comparison. She was one of the first English ships designed specifically for war, and one of the first with big guns mounted inside her hull. She was lost off Southsea on July 19th, 1545, during the Battle of Portsmouth, with the loss of up to 700 lives. The wreck was buried by silt and lay forgotten until her rediscovery in 1836. In 1971 her remains were found again, and after seven years of painstaking excavation, it was realised that the starboard side of the ship was still intact. In 1982 she was raised by the Mary Rose Trust and is now housed in her own museum.

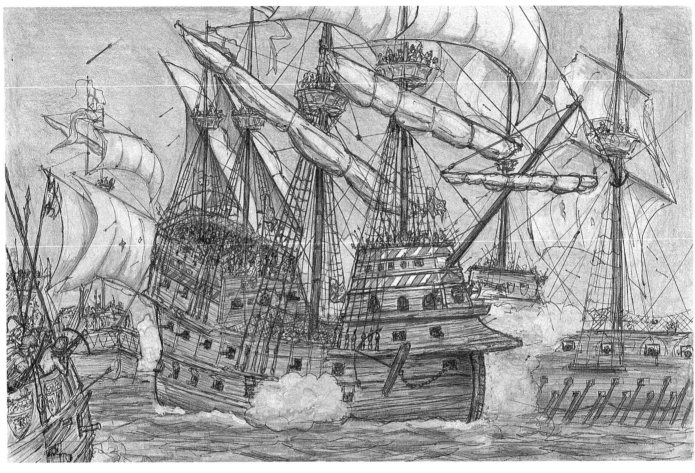

The Mary Rose as she might have appeared going into battle.

The keel of the *Mary Rose* was laid down in 1509, in the final year of the reign of King Henry VII, founder of the Tudor dynasty. Henry had seized the crown from Richard III, last of the Plantagenets, at the battle of Bosworth in 1485. Once established in power, Henry set about recreating a royal fleet of trading vessels and warships. Over the fifty preceding years of weak rule and civil war, the royal fleet had rotted and been replaced by small fleets of converted merchantmen owned by landed magnates. From 1487 Henry ordered the building of several 'great ships.' These vessels were designed specifically for transporting troops and warfare at sea. In 1496 Henry completed at Portsmouth the first dry dock in England. The *Mary Rose* was completed in 1511 at the beginning of the turbulent reign of King Henry VIII. Henry was a warlike king and took a keen interest in his new flagship, which was named after his sister.

She was a large ship by contemporary standards. Her keel was over 100 feet long, with the prow and sterncastle stretching another 50 feet over the water. The hull was 36 feet at the widest with a 16 foot draught and she had a cargo capacity of 700 tons. Much of her weight was carried high above the water line, in the two strong wooden castles built for and aft on the main deck. To propel this heavy load she mounted four masts, two with traditional square-sails and two lateen rigged in the Mediterranean style; about 2,400 square feet of sail. She may seem a clumsy looking ship to modern eyes, but to contemporaries she was beautiful, a potent symbol of the power and majesty of the new dynasty. In 1513 Sir Edward

Howard, the Lord High Admiral, called her "the flower of all ships that ever sailed!"

The young king soon found work for his beloved flagship. She fought in the two French wars of 1512-14 and 1522-25. Naval warfare had changed little in a thousand years. *Mary Rose* was designed to run her prow over the midships of an enemy ship. Then a grappling iron hanging from the bowsprit was entangled in the enemies main rigging, and the two ships locked into a death embrace. High in the masts archers loosed arrows from the five fighting tops. After an exchange of cannon shot, shrapnel, arrows and darts to clear the enemy's decks, soldiers boarded from the forecastle. It was a soldier's battle and knights and nobles, not seamen, were in command.

The crew was clearly divided into separate professions. In 1522 she carried a complement of 426, of these 244 were mariners, 125 were soldiers and archers, 30 were gunners and the remaining 25 servants and trumpeters. Many were skilled professionals. According to Peter Carew half the mariners were capable shipmasters.

When Henry seized the property of the church in 1536 he spent much of the proceeds on naval fortresses and the re-building of his major warships, including the *Mary Rose*. Recent changes in naval design were incorporated. Gunports were cut into her side allowing cannon to be placed on the main deck where they could inflict great injury on enemy ships and high casualties. (Previously guns had been used as anti-personnel weapons or for damaging the enemies rigging). The ship's armament was massively increased. From 1536 she carried 15 beautifully inscribed bronze cannon (including two bronze culverins, 12 feet long and firing large stone round-shot), 57 iron cannon and 70 anti-personnel guns. They were all of different sizes. Thus the *Mary Rose* became one of the first ships with a 'broadside,' giving her the capacity to cripple a ship without boarding, this potential was never realised at the time. The new ship retained its medieval castles, stuffed with guns pointing in every direction. This ungainly mixture of old and new was the key to her eventual fate.

The Battle of Portsmouth

In 1544 the old King's ambitions were aroused and he attacked France, devastating the coast and capturing Boulogne. In 1545 the King of France was free to concentrate his forces for a revenge attack on Henry, he gathered a massive Armada at Le Havre and ordered the Admiral of France, Claude D'Annebault, to capture Portsmouth, Henry's principal naval base and arsenal.

As soon as they knew of the plan, Henry and the Privy Council rode to Portsmouth summoning all available ships and troops. The invasion beacons flared along the coast and the county militias were mustered. Despite these preparations when the French Armada dropped anchor off St. Helens on July 18th, 1545, Henry only had 105 ships to oppose their 235, and apart from his mercenaries there was only a part-time army of militia to oppose D'Annebault's ten thousand professional soldiers. However the English fleet was well equipped and occupied an excellent defensive position. Furthermore, D'Annebault's great flagship the *Carracon* had burned to the waterline at Le Havre, and the night after dropping anchor off Bembridge his new flagship *La Maitresse*

aboard. This extra weight of men and armour high in the castles caused the starboard list to increase until the unsteady soldiers began to stumble across to the starboard side, along with piles of cannon shot and loose guns. Confusion reigned supreme on the densely crowded decks. Water began to rush through the open gunports and the great ship rapidly began to sink. The 700 men aboard were trapped. Most could not swim and were encumbered by armour. Worse, the decks were roofed with anti-boarding netting. Their cries and screams pierced the morning calm "Up to the very heavens" as one courtier recounted: "And the King he cried out like any maid 'Oh my gentlemen!' Oh my gallant men! Drowned like rattens, drowned like rattens." It was quickly over. Two topmasts showing above the water, and a mere 40 survivors.

It was a terrible blow for the English fleet, but it continued to advance, cannon roaring smoke and flame, but unable to close on the galleys for lack of wind. Then a group of English 'Rowbarges' rushed the galleys and drove them back in disorder. However, the English would not attack without the *Mary Rose*.

As D'Annebault had failed to draw the English from their safe waters he held a hasty council of war, and decided to lay waste to the Island, forcing Henry to commit the fleet, or be totally discredited in the eyes of his subjects. The French commanders decided to split the Island's forces by landing at Seaview and Bonchurch, with the main attack on Sandown. The Island's forces under Worsley were mostly drawn up around Yaverland, with weak forces in the East Wight, and some companies of the Hampshire militia guarding the south. When the attack began Seaview and Nettlestone were conquered and put to the flame, and after a bloody fight the Hampshire men were routed, but the main French force was driven back to its boats, both commanders

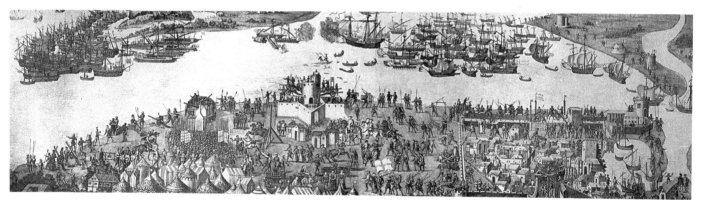

The Battle of Portsmouth from the Cowdray engraving. The topmasts of the Mary Rose can be seen poking above the waves in the middle of the picture. (Courtesy of the Mary Rose Trust).

went aground and sank. In an age of superstitious men these were bad omens.

On the morning of the 19th the sun rose bright over a clear, windless sky. The great French fleet lay at anchor, a colourful display of every kind of oared and sailing warship, decorated with the embroidered banners of half the French nobility. On the Island about 2,000 militia leaned on their pikes and bows and awaited the attack. In Portsmouth the warships were being loaded with extra troops, with the main army being drawn up on Southsea Common. Henry took his place in the newly completed Southsea Castle.

To draw the English fleet away from their sheltered anchorage a group of galleys skimmed across the flat blue Spithead, the sound of their cannon echoing across the water. The two English flagships, the *Henri Grace a Dieu,* and the *Mary Rose,* slid majestically from their moorings to meet them, every sail unfurling to catch the light airs. The *Mary Rose,* under the command of Vice Admiral Sir John Carew, was leading the left wing. When passing close to Southsea Castle she began to list to starboard and swing off course. The mariners were unable to shorten sail and right the ship. It is possible that many were sick with dysentery but confusion is the likeliest cause of their failure. Carew's uncle passed in another ship and called out to his nephew to find out what the problem was. Not being a mariner, Sir George replied "I have the sort of knaves I cannot rule." In fact the mariners could hardly manage the ship thanks to the extra 315 soldiers and archers who had just been put

wounded. The Islanders then marched north towards the smoke clouds that rose from Bembridge where more Frenchmen had disembarked and were pressing inland. Worsley caught the enemy on Culver Down in a charge that drove them almost back to the sea. After a see-saw battle that lasted the rest of the day the French finally withdrew. The Island was saved, as was Henry's reputation, and perhaps Portsmouth itself. A few days later the French sailed off to Boulogne, and the King returned to London leaving orders that the *Mary Rose* should be raised immediately.

Two Venetian engineers were hired and they placed two large ships each side of the Mary Rose and attempted to haul her upright and raise her. However the ship was lying too much on her starboard side, and after a few weeks the whole attempt was abandoned. The great flagship was left to sink down through the soft silt onto a bed of London clay. The silt filled part of the hull, while the rest was pulled apart by the strong Solent currents and eaten away by hungry bacteria. Eventually the ship's remains disappeared, either rotted or buried. Her position long ago forgotten, she would still be there if it were not for a remarkable twist of fate.

The Salvage

Three centuries on in 1836, two brothers, John and Charles Deane, the inventors of the diving suit, were working on the wreck of the *Royal George* for the navy. While thus engaged they were appoached by some fishermen who complained that they had lost

11

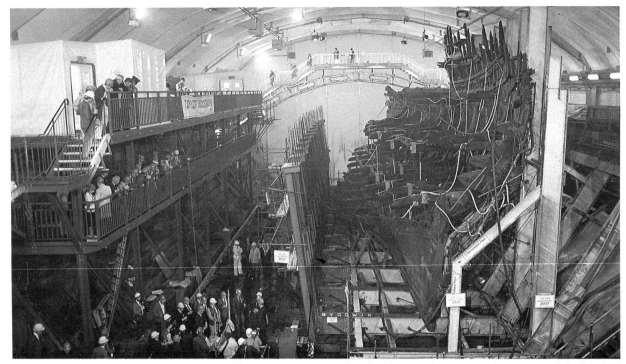

The raised hull of the Mary Rose in the Ship Hall of the Mary Rose Museum after it had been eased into an upright position on July 19th, 1985. (Courtesy of the Mary Rose Trust).

their nets at a certain point off Southsea. The Deanes descended to clear the obstruction and returned to the boat with a bronze Tudor cannon. The *Mary Rose* had been found. A changing current had exposed some of her timbers on which the fishing lines had caught. The Deanes raised four bronze and 19 iron cannon and a number of artefacts from the collapsed port side of the hull. After a short time interest faded and the site was forgotten. For another 130 years the wreck lay at peace in her silt tomb, again lost and forgotten.

The modern story of her salvage begins in the early 1960's when the war historian and diver, Alexander McKee, formed an archaeological diving group who located and explored historic wrecks of the Solent. After several successes, McKee began searching for the *Mary Rose*. In 1966 he read about the Deanes, and taking a hopeful look at some Admiralty charts of 1840, he found the wreck's position clearly marked.

In the following year a committee was formed to find and excavate the ship's remains. Three painfully frustrating years followed. Not a trace of the ship was discovered until 1970, when a cannon was found. It was lying some way from the actual site of the wreck, but it proved that the Deanes were right and this was tremendously encouraging. The following year the first timbers were uncovered.

From this time steady progress was made. The area was mapped with a huge grid and the 'dig' began. Thousands of volunteer divers from all over the world, including H.R.H. Prince Charles, visited and worked on the wreck. Slowly the midships and the remains of the castles were painstakingly excavated. It was discovered that the silt had preserved the timbers of the starboard side and objects aboard in almost perfect condition.

In January, 1979, the Mary Rose Trust was formed to raise and bring ashore the ship's remains. Prince Charles became the President of the Trust. Large funds and much technical assistance was offered over the coming years by individuals and businesses. Between 1978 and 1983 the Trust raised and spent £5,000,000.

Before the hulk of the *Mary Rose* could be raised, she had to be completely and thoroughly excavated and partially dismantled. Over the next three and a half years 3,300 timbers and 16,000 assorted artefacts were raised, requiring no less than 24,640 separate dives.

In late 1982 the Trust was ready to raise the hull. This was a gamble. The ship's soft timbers could not stand much strain. The weather was also a problem, delaying the operation until October, the time of the year when salvage operations are usually abandoned due to the autumnal gales. If the wreck was left another winter, now fully exposed, there may not have been much left of her by the spring.

On October 9th the huge floating derrick *Tog Mor* raised the lifting frame which gently eased the wreck from the mud and placed it on a specially-built cradle on the sea bed. Two days later the whole assembly was slowly raised to the surface. For the first time in 437 years the hull of the *Mary Rose* was touched by the light of day. Then the vast crane of the *Tog Mor* deposited its 500 ton load onto a barge, and the *Mary Rose* made her belated return to base. On December 8th, the cradle and hull were finally placed in Number Three Dry Dock in the Royal Dockyard, next to *H.M.S. Victory,* and close to where she must have been originally built, but this was not the end of the story. The Trust now had to build the museum around the wreck in record time, and it had to be completely insulated from warm air and insects to create the special environment in which the hull could survive. Between February and September nearly 13 tons of aluminium were attached by 97,000 rivets to make an airproof structure covering over 67,000 square feet.

The Ship's Future

If the timbers of the *Mary Rose* ever become dry, they will shrink and crack to pieces. The Trust plans to treat them with a preserving wax but this is expected to take 15 years. To keep her intact until that time she is sprayed with 6,000 gallons of re-cycled chilled water every hour. The air around her must be maintained at a constant five degrees centigrade and 95% humidity. The hull is further soothed by an atmospheric misting system. All the objects saved from her must also be preserved, each particular substance requiring a different treatment.

In October, 1983, the Ship Hall was opened to the public, manned by about 80 volunteers providing guided tours. In May, 1984, the Mary Rose Exhibition was opened in what was No. 5 Boathouse. This show has an excellent display of many of the objects found on board the ship, which allows one to imagine clearly the life aboard a warship built almost 500 years ago, midway in time between the present day and the compilation of the Domesday Book.

In the meantime the Trust has a lot to do. There is the excavation of the crumpled forecastle and other areas around the resting place of the ship in the Spithead. Then there is the study of the artefacts themselves, which has hardly begun; this will slowly reconstruct life aboard the ship in ever increasing detail. There is also more research to be done and of course the long process of preservation and conservation. All this costs money. The Trust needs £400,000 every year to continue its work. In this we can all help by simply visiting the ship and the Exhibition Hall, thus contributing a little more to the greatest archaeological achievement in maritime history.

The Struggle for the Sea Lanes

In the three centuries following the loss of the *Mary Rose,* European mariners explored the oceans of the world in search of trade and coastal and European trade also continued to grow. This led to an increase in the number of wrecks, one of which was a small Dutch ship smashed to pieces under Culver Cliff in 1587. Sir John Oglander wrote that the five crew escaped by climbing the 300 foot cliff, being held against it by the force of the wind. When they reached the top they had to crawl forward on all fours. When the militia sentries saw the five figures crawling over the cliff edge shouting in Dutch they ran for their lives. Later they realised that the intruders were not 'Sea Devils' and carried them down to a nearby cottage where they were cared for until their return to Holland.

Dutch Silver and Spanish Gold

On October 12th, 1627, the Dutch East India Company's autumn convoy set off for India and Indonesia loaded with Dutch silver 'Daalders' and Spanish 'pieces of eight.' On the 14th the little fleet of seven ships was forced by a vicious gale to run for shelter in the Solent. Two of them were so far inshore that they were forced to sail between the chalk stacks of the Needles. The 320 ton *Vliegende Draecke* (Flying Dragon) tore a hole in her bottom and had to be beached, most probably in Alum Bay. The 300 ton *Campen* was less lucky, ending her maiden voyage by grounding and sinking into a shallow grave just south of the middle Needle. Her complement of 160 sailors, soldiers and merchants quickly abandoned her, taking most of the silver. The 200 men and the cargo of the *Vliegende Draecke* did the same, crowding aboard the other ships which soon departed for fear of being seized by the English authorities.

The two ships provided a fantastic bonanza for the Island's salvors and longshoremen. Before the Privy Council had an injunction placed on the wrecks they had been largely stripped and the *Vliegende Draecke* may have been patched up and taken to Yarmouth according to one tale. The following year the *Campen* was worked by a pioneering Dutch salvor, 'Jacob the Diver' and a Newport merchant, Robert Newland. They handed over five cannon, 6,660 kg. of lead and 2,635 coins to the authorities, and going by past experiences probably kept a lot more besides.

The *Campen* was left undisturbed for the next 350 years, she was rediscovered almost by accident by six divers from Northampton, in June, 1979. Teaming up with Richard Larn, an eminent marine archaeologist, to form the Needles Underwater Archaeology Group, they have been working the site since 1980. Despite a difficult swell, visibility of less than a yard and having to use explosives to free the artefacts from the rock, they have raised a number of the possessions of the crew, 103 lead ingots and 8,000 silver coins, no mean achievement.

There are few records for the rest of the century. In 1636, an English treasure ship the *Bird Phoenix*, was wrecked in Compton Bay and in 1691 the English galleon *St. Anthony* was lost in Scratchells Bay, not far from the *Campen*.

In 1688 England and Holland joined forces in a 25 year war against France and Spain. In 1702 their combined fleet was returning from the capture of Gibraltar, when it found the annual Spanish treasure fleet in Vigo Bay. They destroyed the fleet, returning home with five captured gold-laden ships, but at the mouth of the Channel the fleet was scattered by a storm and two of them disappeared. Years later there were many tales of Spanish dollars being found near Blackgang Chine. They were all dated 1701 and were most likely a part of the Vigo treasure. What happened to the ship, its crew and the rest of the cargo remains a mystery.

Trelawney's Treasure

Treasure also featured in the loss of the 44 gun frigate *Assurance*. In 1752 she was sent to Jamaica to bring home Governor Trelawney, who was understandably keen to retire so that he could spend the fortune of £60,000 he had amassed during his tenure. In the soft light of a misty April morning the nine year old frigate approached the Needles, and as was the practice in the Royal Navy, the ship's Master, David Patterson, took over from Captain

Scrope in order to negotiate the difficult passage past the Shingles, which meant sailing close to the outermost Needle. As the jagged mass of rock reared closer Trelawney enquired of Patterson how near they would actually get. "So close that the fly of the ensign (the flag) might touch the rock," he confidently replied. Unfortunately the ship got a lot closer than that, as her keel cracked and splintered on the blackened outcrop of Goose Rock. It is hard to guage how utterly ashamed Patterson must have felt. The 108 foot frigate was a total loss. Boats soon arrived from various Solent ports and Trelawney hired two sloops from Yarmouth to bring ashore his money and help offload the crew. By mid-day the masts had been cut down and the lower decks were awash but Trelawney managed to save all but £4,000 and the crew were all safely landed. Patterson was put away for three months in a debtors gaol. Trelawney was even more unfortunate, after surviving 16 years in disease-ridden Jamaica, he was dead within a year, his fortune unspent.

The Ill Fated Invincible

During the French war of 1756-1763 a much greater naval wreck occurred in the Spithead. This was *H.M.S. Invincible,* originally *L'Invincible,* built at Rochefort in 1744 for the French Navy. She was captured by the British at the battle of Cape Finisterre in 1747.

She was a wonder to her new owners, for though she was a 74 gun 'ship of the line,' she sailed faster than a frigate and yet was bigger than most British 100 gun flagships. During her eleven year service in the Royal Navy she was adopted as a flagship by no less than six admirals, and the dockyard shipwrights used her design for the next generation of British 74 gun battleships. However, the *Invincible* never seemed to accept her new owners, she was dogged by bad luck; on one occasion her masts had to be felled to save her.

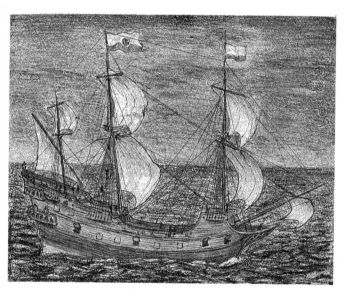

A Dutch East Indiaman of the early Seventeenth Century.

The final disaster struck on February 19th, 1758. The *Invincible* was due to sail with the great military expedition that would conquer Canada from the French over the next two years. As the crew weighed the anchor it snarled and dragged, and after a series of accidents, the great ship drifted aground on Horse Tail Sand. Being heavily loaded with shot and provisions for the long campaign, she proved impossible to refloat. Despite the frantic efforts of vessels from the Spithead, and Portsmouth Dockyard, she rolled over and sank two days later.

She was not rediscovered until one day in May, 1979, when she was found by fisherman Arthur Mack. He teamed up with a local diver, John Broomhead, to set up Invincible Conservations (1744-58) Ltd. which has been exploring and excavating the site since 1980. Among the artefacts raised, preserved, and on display at the Royal Naval Museum in Portsmouth, is a square wooden platter, about one foot wide, from which a seaman would have eaten his regular 'three square meals a day.'

The Back of the Wight in the Eighteenth Century

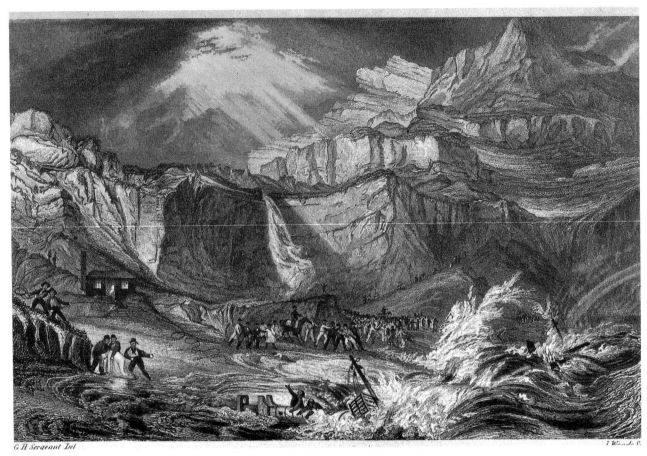

An engraving of a shipwreck at Blackgang Chine

The stormy winters of the eighteenth century proved to be good times for the poor longshoremen of the Island's coasts. While the amount of shipping increased, navigation was still hampered by the lack of sea-going clocks. The result was a steep increase in the number of wrecks. Salvage and the theft of wrecked cargoes became a major local industry closely related to the thriving smuggling trade.

In those days few records were kept but luckily we have one excellent source, the log of James Wheeler, a longshoreman of Blackgang. Begun in 1757, but harking back to 1746, and continuing to 1808, the log records around 110 shipwrecks and one beached whale. In addition to these entries at least 38 other vessels are recorded on the Island's eastern and northern shores between 1740 and 1785, an average of nearly three a year.

Most of these ships were small and were cast high on the beach allowing their crews to escape along ropes. However, there were still many tragedies like the loss of 15 lives in a ship off Rocken End in 1746, or the terrible night of January 10th, 1754, when five ships were wrecked in one night and ten people drowned. The following year the whole crew of a Weymouth sloop died when their ship was torn apart on Rocken End and in November, 1766, a French sloop was smashed to pieces under the chalk cliffs of Freshwater Bay, killing all aboard. In January, 1778, all five crew of a cutter from Alderney died in the cold seas off Brighstone and the whole complement of a sloop 'found eternal rest' at the same place in 1781.

"An Ill Wind . . . "

Apart from these human disasters, shipwrecks were relished by the local people as a providential harvest of wood, work and merchandise. The ships' timbers were used in the construction of houses, boats and sheds; and some of the cargo of most wrecks found its way to the humble cottages of local people. Wheeler carefully recorded the extraordinary variety of cargoes. Spices, salt and sugar enlivened the table to which was added at various times cheeses, fruits, nuts, beans and salted meats. The most common merchandise of the time was alcohol, particularly wines, brandy

and rum. This suited the rough longshoremen (whose drinking habits were legendary), as if they could not drink it all themselves, they could farm it out, along with the enormous range of other goods that fell into their hands, thanks to the smugglers' distribution network.

Wheeler's log shows that the grim rocks of Atherfield Ledge claimed a high proportion of these shipwrecks. On August 12th, 1750, two brigs were cast up on the ledge and another two on the night of January 10th, 1754. Another 19 ships made Atherfield's reefs their final port of call by 1785. Brighstone Ledge also took a heavy toll, becoming known as 'Ship Ledge.'

The end of the American War of Independence re-opened world trade and brought a spate of large shipwrecks. In 1784 two British ships were lost bringing the army back from New York. One was the 750 ton *Earl of Cornwallis,* loaded with army stores and lost on Rocken End. The crew saved a chest containing 7,000 silver dollars but the big ship was lost. Three large American traders were lost on Atherfield Ledge over the next twelve months, all were total wrecks. The last one, the 800 ton *Marchent,* was the third ship ashore in four days.

The First Lighthouses

The sheer volume of shipwrecks made government action essential. In 1781 a number of shipmasters and merchants met in London and drew up a petition which was submitted to Trinity House, the official body responsible for inshore navigation. In 1785 Trinity House began constructing three lighthouses, at Hurst Castle, the Needles and on St. Catherine's Down. The tower at Hurst was lit in September, 1786, but it came to be seen as a failure especially after the loss of *H.M.S. Pommone* in 1811, and in that year it was replaced. The Needles light was constructed on the cliffs 500 feet above Scratchells Bay, the nearest accessible piece of land, and it was often shrouded in mist. The light at St. Catherine's was even less of a success. Soon after building began it was realised that the down was so often buried by cloud that it was almost useless. After costing £7,000 the project was abandoned. Much of the stone was cannibalised for other buildings but the base of this Georgian 'white elephant' still stands, not far from its medieval predecessor.

The Loss of the Royal George

"On the 29th of August, 1782, His Majesties ship the *Royal George,* being on the heel at Spithead, overset and sank; by which fatal accident about 900 persons were instantly launched into eternity." So runs the faded inscription of a Portsea tombstone. It recalls the loss of one of Britain's greatest warships, along with most of her crew and hundreds of Portsmouth people, who were visiting the ship. It is the greatest known tragedy in local history. The causes of the disaster have long been disputed, the Court Martial said that the ship's bottom fell out, when in fact the 100 gun flagship was sunk through the gross incompetence of her officers. Thanks to the false verdict, the salvage attempt of 1783 was consistently blocked by the dockyard authorities and the great ship was left to become a wildlife sanctuary at the bottom of the Spithead.

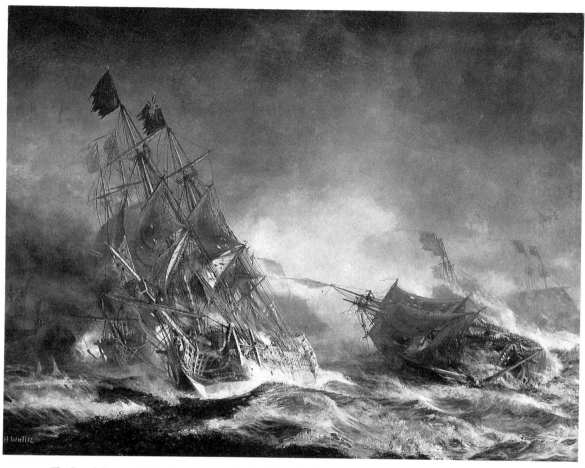

The Royal George sinking the Superbe with a single broadside. "The Battle of Quiberon Bay" by Harold Wyllie.
With acknowledgement to the Royal Navy Museum, Portsmouth.

The story of this fine ship which ended so dismally in the Solent's mud began back in 1746 when the *Royal George* began ten year's construction as the biggest vessel yet built in a British shipyard. On completion she represented the near perfection of the sailing battleship, the development begun so abortively with the *Mary Rose.* As a flagship she was bound to attract the most ferocious attacks so she was built to be bigger, stronger and more powerful than almost any ship afloat. On completion she weighed 3,745 tons. Her hull was over 200 feet long and 50 feet wide while her three gundecks and quarterdeck rose 32 feet above the waves. Her 100 monstrous cannon could deliver one ton of shot with a devastating effect. To resist enemy gunfire she consumed 100,000 cubic feet of English oak and elm.

To propel this massive bulk the ship supported three masts over 100 feet high. Each carried three heavy spars and the intricate cat's cradle of thick tarred ropes and the broad expanse of canvass sail that enabled her to run at 11 knots in a stiff gale.

On the outbreak of the Seven Years War with France in 1756, the *Royal George* took her place as the flagship of the Channel Fleet. Three years later she was given the opportunity to show what she was capable of. In November, 1759, at the Battle of Quiberon Bay, she first knocked out two enemy battleships with only two broadsides despite a gale which prevented the ships using their lower gundecks. Then, as she closed on the French flagship, the 80 gun *Soleil Royal,* the 70 gun *Superbe* bravely sailed between them. The British three decker unleashed her broadside at point blank

range, and the *Superbe* slid beneath the waves. Many more French ships came to the aid of the *Soleil Royal* but the *Royal George* held them off and in the morning the French flagship was beached and burned.

When the war ended in 1763 the *Royal George* was laid up in Plymouth until the new French fleet took to the sea in 1778; in support of Britian's rebelling American colonists. In 1779 a Franco-Spanish fleet occupied the Channel and the British were forced to retreat. The crew of the *Royal George* tied their jackets over the figurehead so that it could not see the ship turning her stern to the enemy. The following year the old flagship redeemed her honour by capturing two Spanish battleships off Portugal. She then began a two year overhaul which brought her back up to scratch among the front line of Britain's navy. In March, 1782, she was declared fit for service and in August she sailed from Plymouth to join a huge fleet being gathered in the Spithead for the relief of Gibraltar.

How Not to Heel a Ship

On the morning of August 29th the calm blue waters of the Spithead were crowded with the hull's of the greatest fleet yet to leave Britain's shores; the view obscured by a forest of masts and spars. Between two and three hundred merchant ships and over 50 "men of war" were loading their final stores. Among the 36 battleships were 6 three deck monsters of which the largest were the *Victory* and the *Royal George.*

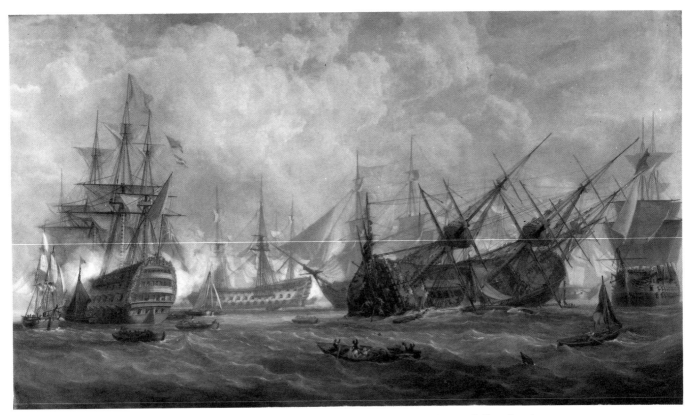

The Royal George capsizing. "The Loss of the Royal George" by Schetky. The Tate Gallery, London.

Before they set sail, Captain Waghorn of the *Royal George* ordered a minor repair to be made below the waterline. A water-cock that provided seawater for cleaning the gundecks needed to be replaced. This hardly interested the ship's nominal commander, Rear Admiral Kempenfelt, even though he had been given strenuous warnings against it by his old colleague William Nichelson, whom he had visited the day before. Nichelson was the Master Attendant of Portsmouth Dockyard and he had told Kempenfelt that to lean or 'heel' the ship while it was loaded with 548 tons of stores and 83 tons of ammunition would be difficult. He also objected to Waghorn's proposed method, running out the port guns and pulling back the starboard guns. In an emergency it would take time to right the ship. Maybe Kempenfelt was not interested or perhaps he felt that the detailed running of the ship should be left to the Captain. In either case he took no part in the heeling operation and gave no instructions to Waghorn. That morning found him working in his cabin.

Waghorn's Blunders

At 7 a.m. the drums rolled and the 820 strong crew began to haul and push the cannon into position. Each one weighed over two tons. The Carpenter and the dockyard plumbers descended the starboard side on a platform. As the ship was so heavy, more guns and shot had to be moved until the starboard list reached eight degrees.

What is extraordinary about Waghorn's decision to heel the ship on the 29th was that that day had been put aside for the crew to make their farewells. In those days seamen were not allowed ashore in case they deserted, so the town came to them instead. Over the next two hours about 360 people arrived in 'bumboats' either to see loved ones or to buy and sell. Soon the upper gun decks were crowded with prostitutes, tinkers and hawkers, wives and children. There was a drunken carnival atmosphere. On such occasions the officers usually accepted that the ship was 'out of discipline.' This not only made it hard for the crew to react quickly to a crisis but meant that a total of 70 tons of humanity was carousing high above the waterline of a finely balanced ship.

The officers made two more gross blunders. No one was in charge of the operation below decks. Despite a fleetwide ban on shore leave, three specialist officers vital to such an operation, the Master, the Boatswain and the Gunner were in Portsmouth. Waghorn and his lieutenants were all chatting in a loose group on the quarterdeck. Furthermore, although the portside gun ports

were less than a foot from the sea Waghorn continued to allow them to be used to load the ship's final stores from a succession of sloops and cutters. The officers also forgot the double flood tide of the Spithead, where the incoming tide from each end of the Solent meets causing a choppy effect, despite the lack of wind. Water began splashing in all along the lower gundeck. From 8 till 9 the wash around the guns grew, and began to splash down into the holds and bilge.

By 9 a.m. the ship's weight had increased by a number of tons, lowering her still further in the water. The ordinary seamen assumed that the officers knew what they were doing, but some, like Quarter Gunner William Murray were getting worried: "I was very uneasy. The water inside was nearly level with the water out."

The Final Straw

At 9 a.m. the 50 ton cutter *Lark* came alongside and began offloading barrels of rum through the gunports. A large number of men were engaged in swinging them aboard and rolling them up the sloping deck but as they were not being organised many of the barrels were simply stacked as they came aboard. This extra weight of rum and men was the final straw, the gunsills were now pulled down below the waterline.

At length the Carpenter noted the danger and hurried to the deck to tell the officers to 'right ship.' As he could not tell who was the duty officer he mistakenly picked the short tempered Lieutenant Hollingsbury, who rebuked the Carpenter and sent him below. This only reinforced the Carpenter's fears and he returned to the deck to repeat his request. "Damn you Sir!" Hollingsbury is said to have replied: "If you can run the ship better than I you had better take command!" Some way off, the returning ship's Master saw the danger and urged his boatmen to full speed. At last the Carpenter warned Waghorn but he merely sent the First Lieutenant to investigate. It was 9.18. The ship had been sinking for 20 minutes and the officers had still not realised the danger. At this point the workmen on the platform cried out: "Avast! Avast heeling! She is high enough. The ship is rising out of the water!" The *Royal George* had begun to capsize. At this point Waghorn ordered the ship to be righted. In a moment hundreds of anxious men were tumbling down hatchways to get to the guns. However, the slope was now so steep that even 18 men could not even begin to move a single gun. "The water began to run in at nearly all the ports on the larboard side of the lower gundeck," recalled one Jack Ingram. There was a frantic panic to get out through the starboard ports but the ship capsized too quickly. Only three escaped through Ingram's porthole.

1,200 People Pulled Down

Up on deck Waghorn dashed to the Admiral's cabin but the door was jammed. The Duty Officer, Lieutenant Durham recalls: "Looking aloft I saw that the masts continued to fall over and I heard Lieutenant Richardson exclaim: "It's all over but I must save this coat!" Following his example I pulled off my coat and leapt overboard." Turning to a young midshipman Waghorn said: "Pierce can you swim?" "No" the lad replied. "Then you must try" said Waghorn and threw him overboard. Both survived but Waghorn lost his own son.

In a few panic stricken seconds the *Royal George* had sunk, pulling 1,200 people down with her. Most were trapped between decks fighting one another for dear life. "The men caught hold of each other 30 or 40 at a time, and drowned one another, those who could not swim catching hold of those that could." Durham was twice pulled down by a marine "who I shook off by tearing my waistcoat loose by which he clung." The marine was washed up a fortnight later with the waistcoat still wrapped around his arms.

The neighbouring ships put out their boats immediately and after the tumult had abated, set about rescuing the exhausted survivors. Many clung to the rigging of the three topmasts which now stood upright above the water. One small boy saved himself by clinging to a sheep, part of the ship's stores. As he did not know his parent's name the man who rescued and adopted him called him John Lamb. Some 300 survivors were dragged from the water, about a quarter of those on board. Kempenfelt, the Carpenter and the Master were among those who drowned. Lieutenant Hollingsbury, the man most responsible for their deaths, survived and was later promoted to Captain.

The Aftermath

For some days the bodies continued to wash ashore, as one ship's Surgeon recorded: "Portsmouth and Gosport were in a state of commotion. Almost everyone had lost some relation, friend or acquaintance. Every hour corpses were coming ashore on the beach. Every hour the bell was tolling and the long procession winding through the streets."

The exact death toll will never be known. The court martial recorded 255 survivors from the 821 crew and many others must have taken the opportunity to escape. The vast majority of the civilians perished.

Many of the bodies were washed up at Ryde and were buried near the shore. The graves were destroyed by building developers in the 1840's but a new memorial was opened by Earl Mountbatten on the same site, now the East Esplanade, in 1965.

The court martial, was rapidly convened aboard *H.M.S. Warspite* and had soon fabricated a story more fitting to the navy's reputation than the truth. The five Admirals sitting in judgement on the crew were determined to clear 'brave Kempenfelt' and Waghorn and shifted the blame for the disaster onto the dockyards authority, the Navy Board. They said that the bottom of the ship had fallen out through rot. They called only 13 witnesses of whom only two supported the verdict. A dockyard shipwright said that some of the timbers were rotten, nothing unusual in a ship 26 years old, and a Gunners Yeoman said that he heard a "bodily crack" below the waterline.

The Admirals framed the Navy Board as the culprit because funds for ship repair were often embezzled, meaning that ships went to sea in a dangerous condition. No less than 83 naval ships sank through decay during the American War. Even the Navy Board believed the verdict on the *Royal George* and as a result they sabotaged every suggestion to salvage the great warship.

Whether she was rotten or not the *Royal George* should and could have been saved. She was sat in the middle of the navy's main anchorage, an embarassing and painful reminder, her great useless masts towering above the water, her 100 terrible cannon menacing passing fish.

Salvage Sabotage

The best idea was put forward by William Tracey in 1783. He suggested harnessing the hull and raising it with the tide and the Board was ordered to cooperate with him. However, the Board used every bureaucratic trick to hinder the operation, even supplying Tracey with ships that sank, and eventually they persuaded the Admiralty to drop the idea. Despite the Board Tracey managed to move the wreck 30 yards to the west before the autumn gales stopped work. Through the winter he kept on two ships and their crews, but when he wrote to the Board in the spring

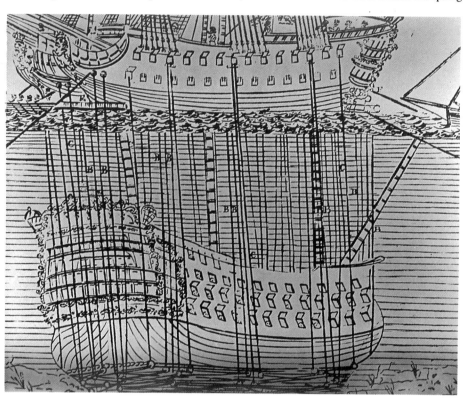

Tracey's attempt to salvage the Royal George in 1783.

they curtly replied that "no further assistance will be given you in respect to your raising the *Royal George*." Bankrupted and crippled through diving, Tracey had the final indignity of seeing his salvage method adopted by the navy without compensation or recognition.

In 1832 the Navy Board was finally abolished and work was resumed on the sunken flagship. Between 1836 and 1839 John and Charles Deane, the inventors of the deep sea diving suit raised 29 guns but reported that the hull was now beyond salvage. In 1839 they were succeeded by Colonel Palsey, a pioneer of marine demolition. He raised the remainder of the cannon by pulverising the hull with massive charges of gunpowder. The now obsolete cannon were melted down and provided the bronze and iron capital at the base of Nelson's Column. Most of the shattered wreck still lies in the mudbank that formed around it.

From Bonaparte to Victoria: 1785-1840

Between the building of the lighthouses of 1785, and the opening of St. Catherine's Lighthouse in 1840, about 75 ships are recorded as being lost around the Island's shores. It was an eventful period that saw Britain become the 'Workshop of the World,' and controller of the world's oceans and trade which meant more shipping and more shipwrecks.

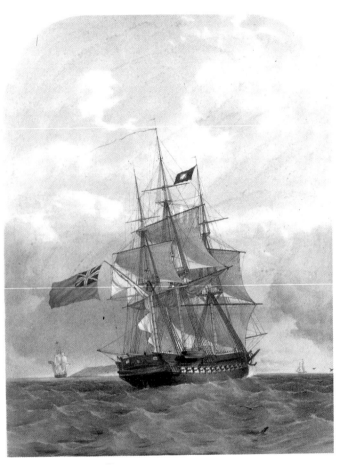

The frigate H.M.S. Pomone, stranded on the Needles and completely destroyed in a few days. The National Maritime Museum, London.

Between 1785 and the outbreak of war with France in 1793 the Channel was busy with 22 ships recorded as coming ashore. The biggest of these was the 900 ton *Juno*, a Dutch frigate of 36 guns and a crew of 250 which was homeward bound from the East Indies. She was wrecked at Sudmore Point on December 9th, 1786 during a violent south-easterly storm. Six of her crew were drowned getting ashore and the ship was a complete loss. Her cargo of "Handkerchiefs, pieces of silk, clothes, money and other things of great value" was completely lost. The remains of the wreck were sold off for £444.

War with France

The war with revolutionary France which began in 1793 became a struggle for world mastery lasting 22 years in which time European trade was strangled by economic blockades, reducing the number of shipwrecks. Wheeler's log recalls a score of ships lost in the early part of the war and then none except warships after 1804. One beneficial wreck was a big ship from Ireland lost on 'Shipledge' in 1795. "A great quantity of oats was sold at 7d a quarter for she remained for some time before she came to pieces."

There were two large wrecks in the winter of 1798-99. The first was a homeward bound East Indiaman, the *Henry Addington*, which ran onto Bembridge Ledge in a thick fog. Unfortunately there was a heavy groundswell which broke up the big ship, drowning 10 or 14 of the crew. Even more dramatic was the loss of the West Indiaman *Three Sisters* in January. She was caught in a violent lightning storm from the south-east while attempting to reach Portsmouth. The crew was lashed by driving snow and rain. The ship went aground on the rocks of Puckaster Cove on the south coast, drowning three of the crew.

Apart from a military transport lost off St. Catherine's in 1800 with the loss of nine lives, the largest loss of the second phase of the war was the 38 gun frigate *H.M.S. Pomone,* wrecked in 1811.

The Sad End of H.M.S. Pomone

The *Pomone* was built in 1805, the year of Trafalgar. She weighed 1,076 tons and was manned by 284 men. She was sent to the Mediterranean where she fought successfully in a series of actions under her able and courageous Captain, Robert Barrie. His greatest triumph was at the Battle of Sagone Bay when the *Pomone* lead three frigates into the Corsican harbour to take on two anchored French frigates and an armed merchantman supported by a fortress and shore artillery. At the days close the fort was silenced and the three French ships were burned to the waterline.

In 1811 Barrie was ordered home to repair his battle-scarred frigate, and while doing so picked up the British ambassador to Persia, Sir Harford Jones, and some Iranian steeds, a present from the Shah to King George III. However, Jones had a more vital cargo, secret intelligence from Sardinia which had to reach Westminster as soon as possible. On the return journey Sir Harford "repeatedly expressed the greatest desire to be back in England as soon as possible." As a result, when the *Pomone* arrived off Portland on October 11th, Barrie set a course through the narrow and treacherous Needles Channel, and handed over command to the ship's Master, James Sturrock. Barrie thought that Sturrock was going to pass too close to the chalk stacks and said to Sturrock: "You must starboard the helm." "If we do that sir, we'll strike the Shingles," Sturrock replied. Barrie went forward to get a view clear of the dense matrix of rigging. Through the mist he perceived Hurst Lighthouse and shouted back to Sturrock: "The light is open by God!" and ran back to the poop to drag Sturrock forward to see the oncoming rocks for himself. The wheel was spun to starboard but it was too late. Two minutes later the *Pomone* struck Goose Rock with a jolting crash.

There was little hope of refloating the ship. She had struck at high tide and was severely damaged. Luckily the sea was calm. When the crew humbly approached Barrie and requested to cover the figurehead in black cloth he finally accepted that his beloved ship was a total wreck.

The Shah's Horses Saved

At midnight the first cutters arrived from Yarmouth and began off-loading the ship's crew and valuables. A marine, Private Lowry, was assigned to the pumps but when he heard an officer say: "It's hopeless" he assumed that his time had come and abandoned his post to get mindlessly drunk with a keg of grog. When he finally appeared on deck, wearing one of the passengers' clothes, his pockets laden with stolen money, almost the whole crew had already gone. He began to babble at Barrie who he thought was someone else. Barrie was not in a mood to listen and ordered Lowry into a boat, but the marine persisted until Barrie had him bodily removed. The evacuation was completed at 2 a.m. but the following day Barrie returned to oversee the salvage operation. Between 30 and 40 small ships bustled around the great wreck, cutting down her masts and carrying away her guns in a hectic race against time. The Shah's horses were somehow manhandled out of a gunport. For three days the salvage continued, becoming progressively more difficult. The groundswell rolled onto the settling ship regularly "spouting to a great height" and running out at the ports. Barrie left the *Pomone* for the last time on the 15th. "The loss of the ship is almost more than I can support." He was relieved of any responsibility for the ship's loss by the Court Martial. Sturrock was severely reprimanded and Lowry was sentenced to 50 lashes of the 'Cat of Nine Tails,' but he was reprieved by Captain Barrie who felt the sentence was unneccesary.

In 1969 the remains of the *Pomone* were rediscovered by a local diver, Derek Williams. The site has been explored over the years by the Isle of Wight County Archaeological Centre. A considerable number of objects have been recovered and are awaiting premises to be made available for a display.

The Carn Brae Castle

Following the peace of 1815 the seas around the Island were again busy with ships and the pre-war pattern of frequent shipwrecks returned. Scores of vessels grounded on the coast every year, most escaping or too small to notice. One unusual case was the loss of the naval schooner *Nightingale,* which was stranded on The Shingles while taking a mad lieutenant to Portsmouth. The crew abandoned him to perish with the ship.

The greatest wreck of the 1820's was the full rigged East Indiaman *Carn Brae Castle,* driven ashore on July 5th, 1829. She had been bound for Bengal with a cargo of manufactures and stores for the East India Company, and a number of company employees and their families. She was driven ashore in a freak summer storm which split her hull on the gnarled rocks of Brook Ledge and forced the crew to saw down the main and mizzen masts. The following morning found the ship listing and low in the water. The swell was too big for the local fishing boats but Coastguard Lieutenant Dornford managed to reach the battered vessel in the Coastguard's cutter and rescued the passengers. Captain Barber decided to stay on to try and salvage the valuable ship.

A small boat was launched to drop an anchor to seaward but it was swamped and the ship's sailmaker drowned. The storm continued, forcing Barber to fell the foremast, and when the gale finally eased the ship was a total wreck. A fleet of small ships came to salvage as much of the cargo as was possible before she completely disappeared.

Lieutenant Dornford's part in the rescue saved his skin in 1836 when he was accused of collusion with smugglers including once ignoring signals for reinforcements during a gun battle between coastguards and smugglers in Totland Bay. He was obviously guilty but his senior officer was bombarded with letters from the Island's gentry and clergy recalling the *Carn Brae Castle* rescue; and

Dornford was acquitted. That same year the ship's remains were the first to be explored by the Deane brothers in their newly invented air-filled diving suits.

The Rocket Apparatus

Just as the Deane's diving suits opened up a new era in marine salvage, another invention transformed inshore sea rescue, the rocket apparatus. The idea of attaching a rope to a projectile and firing it at a shipwreck with a cannon became practical in 1812 when Captain Manby saved 90 people with his rope-firing mortar. In the late 1820's a Carisbrooke antiquarian, John Dennett, tried to adapt Manby's mortar to a rocket, an eccentric weapon that had just been dropped by the army.

The idea was not new but Dennett was the first to build a working prototype, an eight foot cylinder which launched a 23 lb. projectile up to 250 yards. It was stationed with the coastguards at Atherfield.

On October 8th, 1832, the 430 ton *Bainsbridge* was cast ashore on the rocks of Atherfield Ledge and began to break up. The sea was too heavy to launch a boat so Manby's mortar was tried. Four times it fired into the gale but each time the wind was too strong. Then Dennett's rocket was set up and fired. It reached the wreck at the first shot. The line was attached to the ship and fixed to the coastguard's galley, which was hauled out to the wreck with two officers aboard. In two trips they rescued all 19 men from the broken vessel. They later received Silver Medals from the Royal National Lifeboat Institution, formed eight years previously in 1824.

In 1834 Dennett's Rocket was adopted by the Board of Customs and four were stationed on the Island. Dennett continued working on the rocket until his death in 1852, trying to solve the problem of inadequate propulsion which would be finally resolved by Colonel Boxer in 1865.

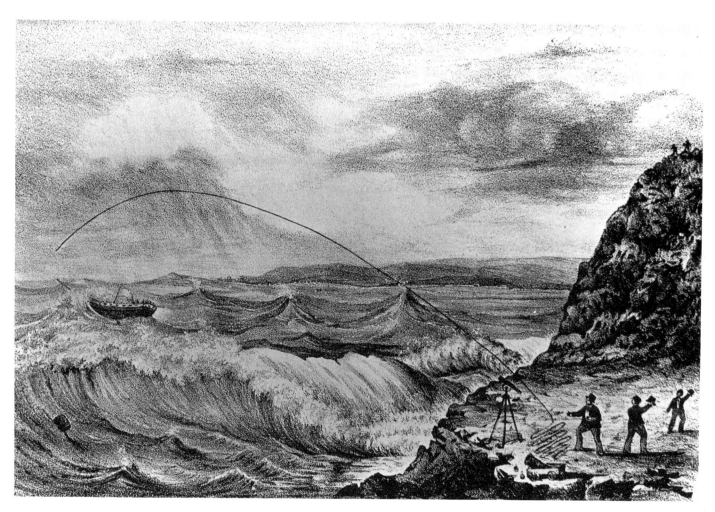

Dennett's Rocket being used for the first time to save the 19 crew of the Bainbridge. Note Manby's mortar in the foreground, the predecessor of the rocket.
(Raymond V. Turley).

The Clarendon Disaster - October, 1836

The most stirring tragedy among shipwrecks along the Back of the Wight was the destruction of the full rigged West Indiaman the *Clarendon*. She came ashore at Blackgang Chine and was quickly demolished by four huge seas. Only three crewmen were saved. Thirteen sailors and ten passengers perished, including two women and five girls. The tragedy transformed the attitude of the local people and as a direct consequence a new lighthouse was built at the base of Rocken End. The new St. Catherine's Lighthouse was opened just 3½ years after the tragedy that inspired it.

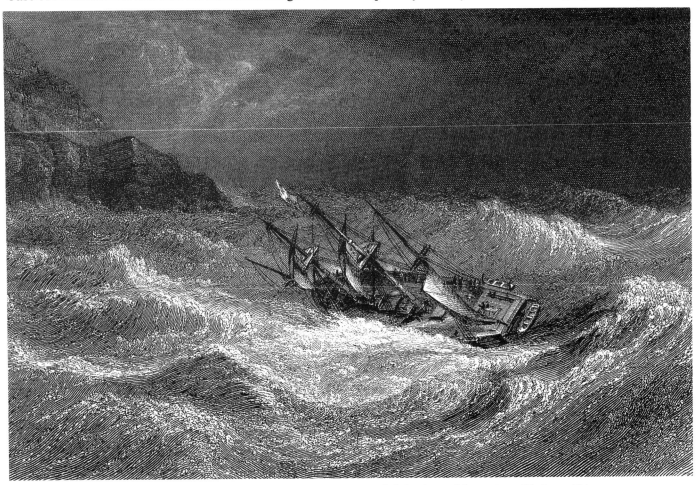

An engraving of the Clarendon being driven towards the shore shortly before her total destruction at Blackgang Chine.

The *Clarendon* was a fine vessel by all accounts, a three-masted ship of 345 tons with a crew of 16 under Captain Walker. She set sail from St. Kitts in the West Indies on August 28th, 1836, with an exotic cargo of rum, sugar, arrowroot, coconuts and turtles. She also carried ten passengers, Captain and Mrs. Shaw and their four daughters, a planter and his 12 year old daughter, a Devon man and Miss Gourley of Portsmouth.

The ship had a rough passage across the Atlantic with strong winds all the way, arriving off Lizzard Point on October 6th. On entering the Channel the winds increased further, forcing Captain Walker to make for the shelter of Plymouth Sound but without success, the ship was driven back out to sea by north-westerly gales and made instead for Portsmouth under close reefed sails. The gale force winds and poor visibility left Walker ignorant of his position.

Mountainous Seas

On the evening of the 10th the gale rose to "hurricane force" generating a huge swell which dwarfed the full rigged ship and reduced the visibility further through spray and rain being thrown horizontally against the straining rigging and the exhausted crew. All through that terrible night the seamen fought to keep the ship under control. The grey mountains of brine broke right across the *Clarendon's* decks and she began to take on board "immense quantities of water." The young girls must have been terrified, but worse was to come.

In the pre-dawn dusk of October 11th the crew saw the south-west coast of the Island and realised they were embayed, with storm force Atlantic winds driving the ship with violent gusts

towards the shore. People on shore saw the big ship struggling in the tempest. In the 1890's Stanley Cotton recorded the verbal account of Mr. Holden, one of the last living eye witnesses, who was only a lad at the time. "The sea was runnen' mountains in the Bay," recalled Holden. The ship "was a'most on her beam ends an' zimmen likely to capsize as each sea struck her." Holden and his father and a number of others began to run along the galeswept cliff top, following the ship and trying to guess where she might come ashore. Captain Walker was still confident that the could weather Rocken End but the winds swung to the south and increased in their fury. The *Clarendon's* fate was sealed but still she fought on. She beat a little to the windward but was pushed back inshore by the mighty white-capped breakers and the gusting wind. The ship pressed on down the coast, somehow missing Atherfield Ledge. There was now only one place where the Islanders could offer any help, Blackgang Chine, otherwise, in that sea, everyone aboard was doomed.

When the fishermen saw it would be Blackgang they sprinted down the wet cliff path to the shore led by John Wheeler, a tall strong ex-naval man. Wheeler dashed to one of the fishermen's huts and grabbed a rope which he tied around his middle and ran towards the deafening roar of the sea. The Holdens were still running along the cliff top when the ship struck. "We didden see her strike but we heard the crash above the storm. It sounded like a box bein' stove in but hunnerds o' times louder. Father groaned and I started to sob."

John Wheeler followed the retreating sea to about 30 yards from the crumpled ship and yelled and waved at the people to jump. One did and Wheeler grabbed him and the two were washed in by the next sea with those on shore hauling on the other end of Wheeler's rope. Without a second to lose Wheeler rushed back still shouting into the tempest, the masts tearing and falling just a few yards from where he was wading back to the ship. He grabbed another man, and another sea smashed through the ship, swamping the screams of those on board.

Terrified Cries For Help

The fourth wave demolished the ship completely. When the Holden's reached the beach "The ship was gwyne to pieces and we could see many of the people strugglin' in the water. Their terrified cries for help pierced our very souls. Father and me grabbed the rope just as John was draggen the third man through the surf. Then a tremendous wave knocked 'em both down and we aveared they'd be sucked back by the undertow. But we hauled like madmen, and at last they came ashore."

Wheeler saved the only three survivors, the second mate and two seamen. Everyone else died in the sea, their bodies broken and crushed by the ship's timbers which "lifted to the waves like so many trees." Young Holden staggered away from the scene like a man who was drunk, to the sound of the ship's piano smashing on the rocks "the awful clang! clang! . . . It was the Devil's music surely." His father and others remained on the beach to pick the naked mangled bodies of the ship's company from the surf. They were carried up to the church. At the sight of the bare broken bodies of the Shaw girls the hardened old fishermen began to weep.

The village of Chale was in deep shock. "I shall never forget the look on the faces of everybody I met . . . nobody thought of any meals or much else . . . we just moved about like folk out of their senses."

Captain Walker and most of the others were buried under the north wall of the graveyard at St. Andrews and were provided with modest headstones. One body did not come ashore, that of Miss Gourley. The sea carried away her body and deposited it at Southsea, at the foot of her father's garden.

By another uncanny coincidence one of the men that Wheeler rescued, Thomson, turned out to be an old shipmate. They had both served on Lord Yarborough's yacht, the *Falcon,* and four years previously Thomson had saved Wheelers life, so now the score was even. Wheeler continued to distinguish himself in rescues. The following February he carried out an identical rescue of three men from the French lugger *Jean Marie,* for which he received the Silver Medal from the Royal National Lifeboat Institution.

The Legacies of the Clarendon

In honour of the dead the White Mouse Hotel at Chale became the Clarendon Hotel. The Clarendon Hotel in Shanklin was built with the timbers from the ship, as were many houses in the Chale area.

The greatest legacy of the lost lives of the *Clarendon* is St. Catherine's Lighthouse. For centuries Island people had been complacent about a light at St. Catherine's Point, one of the greatest hazards in the Channel. Wrecks brought great advantages for salvage and theft but the *Clarendon* tragedy changed all this. Trinity House was stung into action by repeated local demands for a lighthouse, and construction began in the following year.

To avoid the old problem of hill fog the 107 foot tower was built at the foot of the cliff on Rocken End, the base being just 72 feet above sea level. This position allowed it to shine along the treacherous southern coast, into Chale Bay and deep into the English Channel.

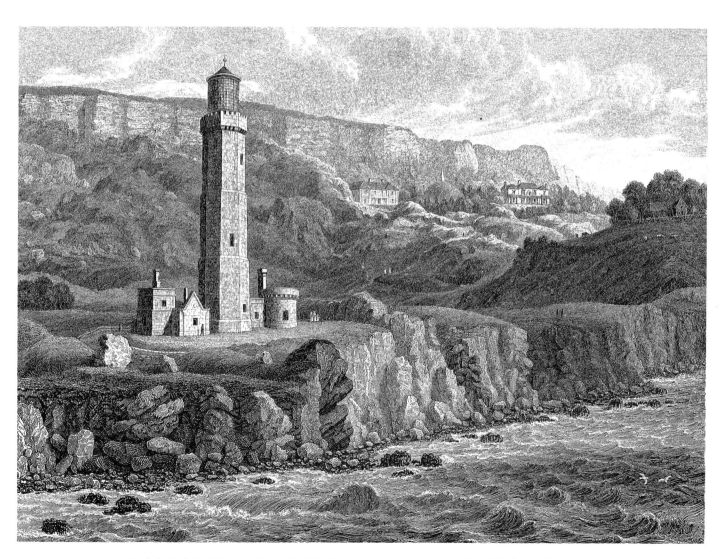

St. Catherine's Lighthouse as it looked originally. An engraving by Brannon. (The I.W. County Press).

Lighthouse and Coastguards: 1840-1860

Between March 1840, when St. Catherine's Light began operating, and early 1860, when the first lifeboat stations were being organised at Brook and Brighstone, there was a marked development in the Island's sea rescue services. The Coastguard became increasingly involved in saving life from shipwrecks and in 1859, the new Needles Lighthouse was completed. Nevertheless, this period saw its share of violent storms and some of the worst tragedies of the century.

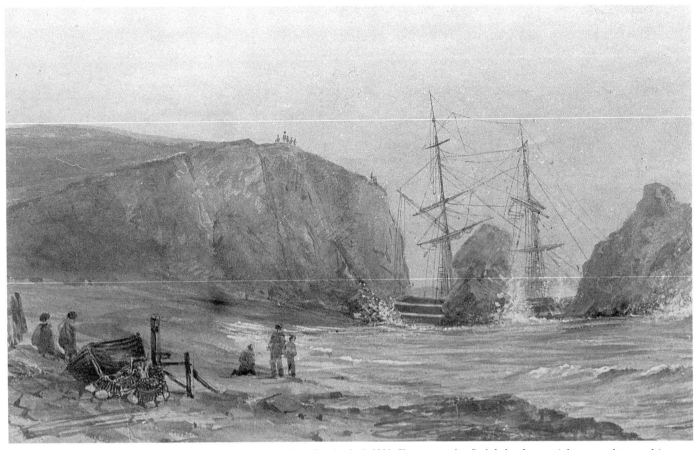

The Norwegian brig Perlen striking Stag Rock in Freshwater Bay, October 2nd, 1851. She attempted to find shelter from a violent storm but was driven ashore becoming a total wreck. Sandpainting. (Courtesy of the Trustees of Carisbrooke Castle Museum).

The Eighteen-forties and fifties continued to see a number of ships ashore with every winter gale. During a single storm in January, 1843, two vessels foundered in the Spithead and four more were cast ashore between Stokes Bay and Hayling Island. The brig *George*, bound for Grenada in the West Indies, was driven onto the ugly teeth of Atherfield Ledge and was torn apart. The Captain and Mate were swept away but the remaining 11 crew were saved by the rocket apparatus attaching a line along which a boat was able to reach the dying ship.

Two years later the Yarmouth coastguard cutter saved six men from the barque *Siam*, stranded and breaking up in Compton Bay. The rest of the ships crew had made it ashore in one of their own boats. Coastguard Lieutenant Gould received the R.N.L.I. Silver Medal.

In 1848 another large sailing ship, the *Llanrumney*, drove onto the rocks at Atherfield with 15 men aboard. Two fishermen, heroes of the *George* rescue, put out to her in one of their boats but it capsized in the breaking seas and they were both drowned. Then Lieutenant Bulley, leader of the *George* rescue, organised another volunteer crew and saved everyone aboard the ship. For this and other rescues Bulley became the most decorated coastguard in the Island's history, with the Gold Medal and Bar and two Silver Medals.

The bravery shown by Bulley and many other coastguards began to win the respect of the local people who at first hated the service. The coastguard had originally been established in 1822 as a paramilitary force designed to defend and police the coasts. Their duties involved crushing the smuggling trade and arresting anyone found picking up shipwreck from the beach. As a result the longshoremen and coastguards were natural and bitter enemies, but as time passed the call to save life and the mutual admiration instilled by each others courage triumphed over the conflict of interests. As time passed smuggling declined and the coastguard became primarily involved in sea rescue.

Brig Ashore in Sandown Bay

A good example of this co-operation is seen in the story of the rescue of 19 men from the Swedish brig *Tale Banre*, which was driven ashore in Sandown Bay during a terrific south-easterly storm. The power of the wind was such that although the ship grounded 400 yards out it was beaten ever closer to the beach, breaking up all the time, her sails torn apart by the wind. Despite the conditions five coastguards and two fishermen put off in the coastguard's whaleboat. Twice it was swamped and driven back to the beach but on the third attempt they reached the tattered brig and saved one man before the boat was swamped again. On the fourth attempt the whaleboat saved six men but was now so badly damaged that it could not be launched again, so three fishermen put out in their own tiny boat and rescued the rest of the crew in four desperately dangerous trips. Their boat was destroyed. In the morning the *Tale Banre* was lying on Sandown beach, no longer a ship, just a mangled heap of wood. Both coastguards and longshoremen could congratulate themselves on a magnificent rescue.

The Abby Langdon

One of the biggest wrecks of the fifties was the *Abby Langdon*, a full rigged American ship loaded with Burmese rice. She was driven onto the rocks on the night of August 9th, 1858, about a mile east of Freshwater Bay. Dawn of the 10th found the ship in a deplorable position, creaking on a mattress of boulders beneath forbidding 300 foot chalk cliffs. She was broadside onto the sea, leaning to starboard and leaking. When the coastguard failed to pull her off at the next high tide Captain Hall realised that his only chance lay in unloading the ship before the rice became wet and heavy, and began to expand. His men managed to offload 3,000 sacks by the following day but it was no good. A strong south-westerly came up, blowing great waves across the wide expanse of Compton Bay. "No barges will come out," lamented the Lloyds agent, but who could blame them, they would be risking their lives as well as their ships on such a lee shore. The *Abby Langdon* settled into her uncomfortable grave and water began to gush into her hold drowning the pumps, and forcing the crew to abandon her. The rest of the cargo and half the ship's stores were lost. Her remains were sold off two weeks later.

The New Needles Lighthouse

While the auctioneer's hammer poised over the *Abby Langdon's* dismal future, just a few miles west, work was nearing completion on one of the greatest achievements of the decade, the new Needles Lighthouse.

The old light, being 500 feet above sea level was often buried under low cloud, and ships continued to drive onto the rocks below with a monotonous regularity. The solution was offered in the plan of the architect James Walker, which suggested building the lighthouse at sea level by dynamiting a platform on the outermost Needle. It was a tough engineering job. The proposed site was exposed to hurricane force winds and waves up to 20 feet high The lighthouse base was stepped to break the waves and the 100 ft. tower was given a granite wall a yard thick at the base, tapering to 18 inches at the top. As the three man crew was likely to be cut off for weeks during the winter, additional cellars and a 2,400 gallon watertank had to be blown out of the chalk. All the materials had to be ferried through some of the most dangerous waters around Britain. In this respect the builders were greatly aided by the Conways, a famous Freshwater family of longshoremen, who acted as ferrymen.

The Tragic Winter of 1859

The lighthouse was completed in 1859, just before one of the worst winters in the Island's maritime history. In just two months four ships were destroyed and fourteen lives lost.

The first casualty was the schooner *Lelia,* which was sailing from Nassau with a cargo of sponges and a crew of seven, when she was caught up in a storm that lashed Britain's coasts for 15 days from October 25th, causing 325 wrecks and 748 deaths nationally. The *Lelia* was cast ashore on Rocken End on November 1st. One of the crew was washed away and drowned but the others were rescued by local men, led by James Thomas, who recieved the R.N.L.I. Silver Medal. The ship was smashed to pieces and scattered for five miles along the coast.

Mirabita Disaster: 11 Drowned

This loss was followed by two more on December 5th during a tremendous south-westerly storm. The first ashore was the *Mirabita,* a barque from Malta, loaded with oats from Marseille and carrying 16 crew. She grounded a mile from the shore on Brighstone Ledge and was soon being swept by the huge angry seas, then running in the bay. The crew could be clearly seen in the rigging by those onshore, but they could not be reached. Every attempt to launch a boat was a failure.

The *Mirabita* was soon joined by the schooner *Sentinel* of Carnarvon, which came ashore further towards Brook. The sea and wind increased in their fury until the big crowd ashore could see that the *Mirabita* was starting to break up. Her masts began to topple, throwing her screaming crew into the maelstrom of breaking waters below. Their cries carried clearly to the cliff on the wings of the gale. Some were struck by pieces of wreck while others gave up the struggle as they were tossed and buried by the breaking waves. Only five gasping survivors were pulled from the surf alive.

It seemed as if the *Sentinel* must suffer the same fate. Two of the crew had already been swept away. The Lloyds agent reported the desperate scene to his paper: "She still holds together, and the crew are seen in the rigging, but at present there is no hope of saving any of them." However, a little later the wind moderated and seven men, led by Thomas Baker, launched a boat from Brook Bay. The Reverend Pellew Gaze of Brook and others waded in up to their waists to push the boat clear over the incoming rush of the sea. The effort was a success. The four survivors aboard the *Sentinel* were brought safely ashore. The following morning their ship had joined the *Mirabita* in a long thick line of pulverised fragments along the beach. Both ships had been annihilated. No one was much interested in the humble pickings along the shore. Brighstone and Brook were in a state of shock, as Chale had been after the *Clarendon* disaster. The cries of the *Mirabita's* crew still rung in their ears.

The last ship ashore that year was the schooner *Jane,* which was wrecked at Blackgang on Christmas Day. The ship was a total loss, but the crew were saved.

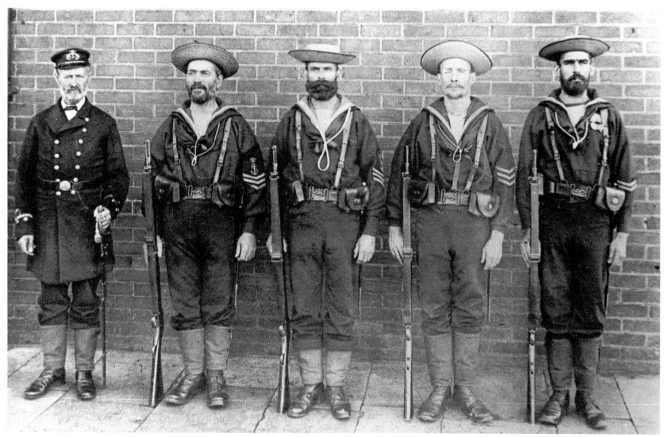

Coastguards on parade at Ventnor towards the end of the Nineteenth Century.

The Coming of the Lifeboats: 1860-1878

The wrecks of December, 1859, had a dramatic effect on Island opinion. In several quarters plans were laid and money raised for a lifeboat to be placed on the exposed west coast. The vicars of Brook and Brighstone formed a committee which raised the extraordinary sum of £600 in two months. In addition, the Royal Victoria Yacht Club raised another £275. These funds were placed at the disposal of the Royal National Lifeboat Institution, which found that it had enough to build two boats at £200 each, construct two boathouses and pay all the costs for a year. It was a good start.

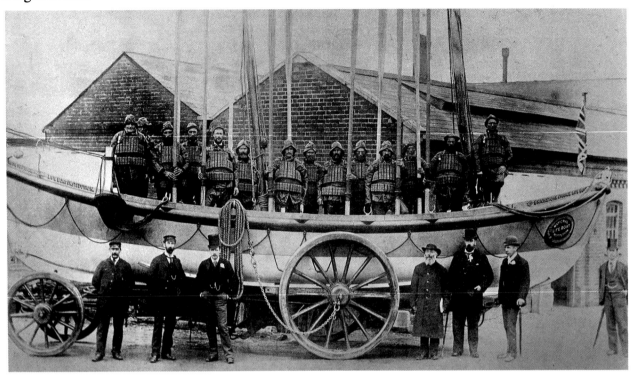

The Brighstone Lifeboat Worcester Cadet with her crew and officials. (Courtesy of Geoffrey Cotton).

In the choice of where to station the two boats, the Institution was limited by geography. The obvious areas were Brighstone and Atherfield Ledges, but 'east of Brighstone no chine was suitable as no horses could be got down to the shore.' So the two boats were placed at Brook and Brighstone Grange Chines.

The two boathouses were quickly completed and on August 13th, 1860, the lifeboats arrived at the villages to simultaneous ceremonies. The volunteer crews unanimously elected their coxswains and the *Rescue* of Brighstone and the *Dauntless* of Brook were taken down to the waters edge. A bottle of wine was broken over each bow by the two most prominent ladies and the crews took the boats out for their first trials. It was a quaint start in a career that would take the two villages to the headlines of the world.

Each boat was 30 feet long with a thick heavy hull and powered by eight massive oars. Later they were adapted to take 10 oars to give the unwieldly boats more power and direction. The basic design of the self-righting boat had been worked out in the 1790's and since refined to make a boat that was self-righting, unsinkable and unbreakable. However, the massive weight of the hull made the boats difficult to launch, row and sail.

" . . . out of the boat you go!"

To launch, the boat was brought down to the waters edge on its carriage, which was pulled by a team of 10 horses along with about 30 launchers and the crew. The operation was well described by General Seely, later Lord Mottistone, in his book 'Launch.' (He was a native of Brook and for many years a member of the lifeboat crew). The carriage was backed into the surf; the crew sat with oars poised; the two lines of launchers stood ready to haul in the lines 'which shoot the boat from the carriage into the sea.' All awaited the coxswain's command.

For a launch to be successful a number of vital conditions had to be met. It had to be into a large long wave with plenty of volume. If the order was given a few seconds early, the boat would be thrown broadside onto the beach by the incoming breaker and capsized. It would take an hour to make it ready again. If the boat

was launched too late it would slide down the back of a wave 'at an incredible speed' and would crash into the beach to be swamped by the next wave. 'No lifelines will hold you then; out of the boat you go!' To launch at the right moment required expert judgement by the coxswain and an instantaneous response from the launchers. To ensure success 'the 10 oars must strike the water at the same moment, the instant the lifeboat is waterborne.' Furthermore, the second stroke had to sweep the water before the oncoming wave. Only then could the lifeboat be launched.

In addition to all this, one must imagine the conditions in which the boats were normally launched. Sometimes it was pitch dark, with waves breaking up the cliff, and with the shouts of launchers drowned by the crashing of the sea or snatched away by the gale. Everyone would be soaked, shaking with cold, and hardly able to see or hear. Such times as these bring out special qualities in people, a determination and super-human strength, combined with instinctive collective action. General Seely noted that even the horses, which must have been petrified "seemed to be imbued with the same spirit, as any carter will tell you." Despite all these conditions, almost every launch was a success.

Unnecessary Tragedy

The first call for the Brook boat *Dauntless* came on New Year's Day, 1861. At 7 a.m. the 32 pounder lifeboat cannon boomed out, and in a few minutes the whole village was alive with activity. The *Dauntless* was soon launched and bound for the 110 ton schooner *John Wesley*. She was anchored in a dangerous position in Compton Bay, but the Captain twice declined coxswain John Hayter's offer of help, and twice the lifeboat returned to shore, even though her crew could see that the schooner was doomed. At 2.30 p.m. the coastguards saw the ship go aground under the high chalk cliffs, they alerted the lifeboat and prepared a cliff rescue. Two coastguards descended to the ship by ropes, they and the lifeboat reached the wreck to find it empty, the crew had boarded a tug and were chugging safely away to Southampton.

All seemed well, but then tragedy struck. While climbing back up the cliff the coastguards were caught in a cliff fall, and one,

Coastguard McLeod, was killed. It was a sadly unnecessary tragedy.

The Convict Ship

On April 2nd, 1862, the Brighstone boat received its first call to the 308 ton barque, *Cedrene* which was stranded on Ship Ledge in thick fog and a heavy swell. The *Cedrene* was a masterpiece of Bermudan shipbuilding, "the loveliest three masted barque ever built," and just 16 days old. She had left Bermuda on March 16th, bound for Portsmouth. At 1 a.m. on April 2nd, her mate mistook the Island for a great black cloud. He called the captain, who ordered the ship about, but too late. The fine ship was soon helplessly driven aground.

When Coxswain James Buckett drew alongside in the *Rescue* he was shocked to find that the *Cedrene* was carrying a human cargo, 191 convicts returning home, their sentences finished, and another 43 overseers and crewmen, a total of 234 people to be safely landed.

In eight trips the *Rescue* brought 134 people ashore, including all the women and children. By this time the groundswell had driven the wreck so close inshore that a line could be attached, along which the rest of the men could make their way through the surf to the beach. The Rev. Pellew Gaze and the chief coastguard, Joe Cutajar, were later commended by the R.N.L.I. for their outstanding gallantry during this beach rescue.

Leaving the massive crowd on the beach, many of the ex-convicts made their way to the two Brighstone pubs to celebrate their return to England, good ale and the fact that they were still alive. Having drunk the pubs dry, some started to fight in the road outside. The inhabitants of Brighstone must have been very relieved by the arrival of troops from Parkhurst Barracks, who marched the offenders off to Newport.

The *Cedrene* itself was a total wreck, left high on the beach by the tide. There she was broken up, her long lasting cedar timbers providing fine material for local buildings, including Mottistone Church, "where the fragrance of Bermuda Cedar still lingers after 100 years . . . a token of the beauty that was *Cedrene.*"

Death at Ladder Chine

On the night of October 20th, 1862, the sky blackened in the west and the wind built up into a tearing gale. The people of the 'Back of the Wight' knew it was wrecking weather and they prepared the lifeboats for immediate launching. Out in the Bay, hidden by the thick rain, two ships were fighting a hopeless battle to avoid being driven ashore.

The first ashore was the barque *Helen Horsfall*, which loomed out of the darkness at Cowlees Chine, near Brighstone, and was quickly aground. There was no time to launch the *Rescue*, but the crowd onshore was able to assist the whole crew ashore, including the Captain's wife and child.

The crew of the East Indiaman, *Lotus,* were not so lucky, no one saw her when she crashed ashore at 11.45 that night, not far from Ladder Chine. Even the coastguards, squinting into the gale at Atherfield Point, only a few hundred yards away, did not see or hear the doomed ship.

The storm was so powerful that the *Lotus* was demolished in a matter of minutes. Only two of the 14 crew survived. Captain MacNeil did not have time to fire the ship's cannon, it all happened so fast.

Ordinary seaman Jim Gold, recalled what happened while giving evidence at the Inquest.

"I was at the wheel, taking orders from the Captain. The sea immediately broke over the ship and knocked the Captain down as he was giving orders to clear away the boats. I think he was washed overboard then, as I never saw him again afterwards. Another sea immediately followed the first and took away the First Mate, the long-boat and the gig. The carpenter jumped into the sea and swam for the shore, got to the beach, but was taken back again by another sea that broke over him. I did not see him again. By this time the masts had gone overboard and the ship had parted below the chains. I clung on to the wreck until three seas went over me, when I got on to a rum barrel and the next sea took me and the rum barrel right ashore, but another took me out again. I was afterwards washed in again and found myself lying among some broken timber and wreck high on the beach."

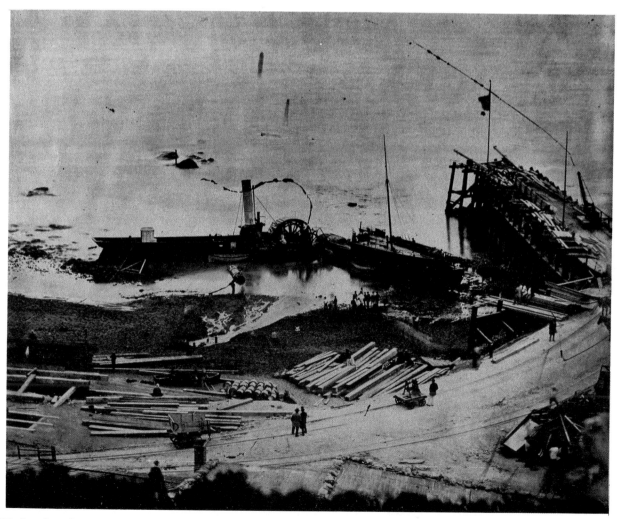

The brand new iron passenger steamer Chancellor stranded and broken in two next to the half-completed Ventnor Pier on July 3rd, 1863.

(Courtesy of Andy Butler and Robin McInnes).

The other survivor, Anderson, came ashore on a spar. A man with him was drowned.

The *Lotus* and her cargo of sugar and rum were scattered in pieces along the shore. The recovered bodies of the crew were buried at St. Andrews Church, Chale.

It was the winter of 1864 when the Brighstone crew were called on again. On January 19th the schooner *Thetis* was struck by huge seas five miles south of St. Catherine's Point and foundered. Her four man crew just had enough time to escape in the ship's boat and attempted to sail it towards the Island, after 12 hours they were seen from the shore. The *Rescue* soon reached the exhausted frozen men and dragged them aboard, their waterlogged boat capsized shortly after they had abandoned it.

The Children's 'Dove'

While the lifeboatmen were scoring their first successes, back on land more money was being raised and more stations established. The Isle of Wight Sunday School Committee raised enough money to build another boat. The children's boat was called the *Dove*, and built at J. Whites, the Cowes shipbuilders, who constructed generations of fine lifeboats. On Coronation Day, 1868, a gay procession of children who had raised the money, escorted the new boat from the boatyard to Cowes Green and then to the sea for her trials. The *Dove* was not an R.N.L.I. boat, she was looked after by a board of trustees. In 1869 they moved her to Totland Bay where a house was built. She remained there for 15 years in which time she saved 36 lives, 17 from the barque *Magellen*, which went down in 1883. In 1885 the Totland Station joined the R.N.L.I. and the *Dove* was housed at a new station at Shanklin. She remained there

until 1917, when she was washed out of her boathouse during a terrific storm and taken away by the sea.

In 1867 the two R.N.L.I. boats were replaced by two new 10 oar boats. The new Brighstone boat was also called *Rescue*, while the new Brook boat was called the *George and Anne*. The following year a new station was set up at Bembridge with the encouragement of the navy, partly as a result of the Nab Light being moved out to sea, and partly because the R.N.L.I. were impressed by the rescue of the crew of the barque *Egbert* by local fishermen in an ordinary open boat. The boathouse was completed in 1867 and the new boat, *The City of Worcester,* arrived in 1868. Next year another independant station was established at Ryde where the *Captain Hans Rusk* was installed to watch over the busy waters of the Spithead.

The Boxer Rocket

Thus by 1870 the Island was well equipped to deal with the increasing volume of maritime traffic around its shores. Apart from the lighthouses, the Island boasted five lifeboat stations and an excellent intelligence and rescue network in the Coastguards, who were now being issued with Boxer Rockets. Colonel Boxer solved the problem of inadequate propulsion by putting one rocket behind another, to act as a booster when the first rocket reached maximum elevation. Combined with the Breeches Buoy, invented by Lieutenant Kisbee, the Boxer Rocket saved over 100 lives on the Island alone before its replacement in the 1950's.

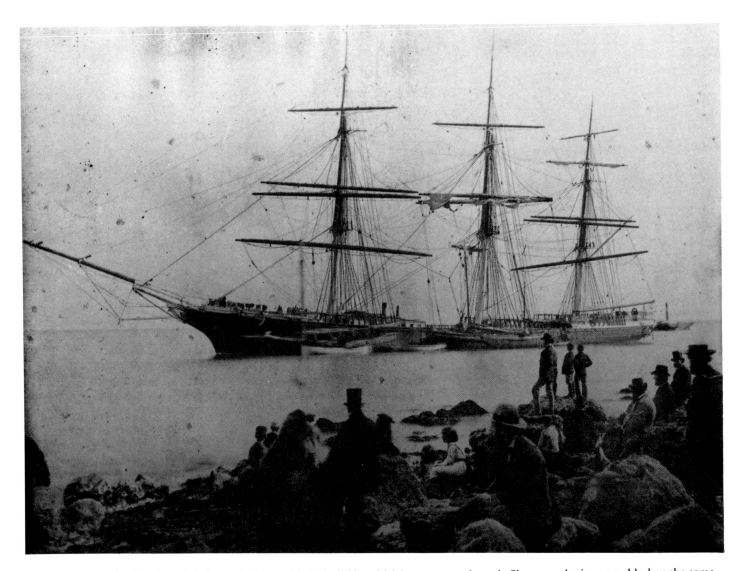

This is the 900 ton *Underley,* a full rigger, the biggest kind of sailship, which became a total wreck. She was only six years old when she came ashore, on a dark night in September, 1871. She was bound for Melbourne with 30 migrant passengers and £30,000 of cotton goods, machinery and gunpowder. The moon went down and a sudden south-easterly pushed her straight onto the rocks between Luccombe and Bonchurch. The crew furled the sails but did not drop the anchors, so the great iron ship swung broadside onto the shore where she could not be saved. In the foreground are the passengers who came ashore in the morning to watch the efforts to tow her off. The crew abandoned the ship the next day, all except the Steward, who was drowned going back to rescue his pet canary. The ship was broken up and soon disappeared.

The Wreck of the Cassandra

In mid November, 1871, the fine Liverpool barque *Cassandra* was sailing to London from Madras when she was caught in 'a particularly fierce westnor'west gale' in the Channel. On the night of the 15th she was driven onto the long rocky fingers of Brook Ledge, in Compton Bay. The Brook lifeboat, *George and Anne,* was brought down to the beach, pulled along it to the wreck and launched. The *Cassandra* was rolling heavily on the ledge but was not in immediate danger. Coxswain Hayter wanted everyone to come ashore but the Captain thought they were safe enough, and the lifeboat returned with only seven of the 21 crew, including the injured. The lifeboat was taken back up the chine and re-housed.

An hour later the *Cassandra* was signalling for assistance. The whole lifeboat launch procedure had to be repeated but now the tide had risen. The seas were breaking right over the wreck and up the cliff, over the exhausted launchers and horses. Nevertheless the re-launch was successful and the remaining 14 men were saved.

Destroyed in Four Days

The next major wreck, the St. Malo brig *L'Etoile,* called out both the lifeboats. She came ashore between the two stations at Sudmore Point, on the night of May 3rd, 1872. 'The night was intensely dark, a fresh gale blowing from the south-west with rain and a heavy groundswell.' *George and Anne* launched straight into the blackened sea at Brook while the Brighstone boat, *Rescue,* was dragged 1¼ miles along the beach and launched directly opposite *L'Etoile* which was in a terrible state. Heavy seas were breaking over her, forcing the crew into the rigging, all eight were saved by *Rescue.* The *George and Anne* arrived 10 minutes later. 'Within four days the *L'Etoile* and her cargo of salt had completely disappeared.'

The Doomed Brigantine Hope

The Island's rescue services could do nothing for the crew of the doomed brigantine *Hope.* In December, 1872, she attempted to find shelter from a furious storm by sailing into Freshwater Bay. According to the Island's Recorder of Wrecks, Holms, the *Hope* struck the outer reef of the bay. It was probably in the hollow of a wave, as she struck hard and went to pieces immediately. Not one of her crew reached the shore alive. 'All on board must have perished instantly, the sea being very heavy.' Only the stern and 'a small fraction of the hull' came ashore.

The First Steamer Ashore

Later that same winter, on February 2nd, the 640 ton steamer *Woodham* got into difficulties in the Channel. She was a Norwegian ship bound from Newcastle to New York with 22 crew. The previous day the propeller shaft had broken, but luckily a Liverpool steamer had taken her in tow. However, the weather turned foul, Lloyds Lists reported strong east-south-easterly winds with rain, sleet and snow. Three times the hawser broke and had to be re-connected, when it broke again, the two ships lost one another in a dense snowstorm. The *Woodham* drifted on, crippled and helpless, until she grounded at Chilton Chine, at two o'clock in the morning.

The crew of the *Rescue* were summoned at 5 a.m., but found the sea so heavy at Grange Chine that they dragged the boat along the beach and launched opposite the wreck. When *Rescue* drew alongside at 7 a.m., Captain Helgesson was preparing to lower his boats. Coxswain Buckett persuaded him to use the lifeboat, and in two trips brought the 20 crew ashore. However, Helgesson and the Mate felt safe enough and stayed on board despite Buckett's advice. The lifeboat returned to Grange Chine and was re-housed. "By now the crew and launchers were thoroughly wet through and cold and were soon on their way up the road to home, but it was not to be, as more distress signals were seen coming from the *Woodham.*" By now the tide was too high to take the lifeboat along the beach. "It was decided to take the lifeboat overland. The crew and launchers, armed now with axes, spades and saws, set off first for about one mile along the old Military Road, then the cutting down of gateposts and widening of the chine were necessary." As they hacked out a path down steep Chilton Chine, the gale-driven snow froze their hands and faces. At last the *Rescue* was manoeuvred to the shore and the second launch attempted, 'under very dangerous circumstances and in terribly severe weather.' The seas were breaking over and into the great iron ship. As soon as the *Rescue* got close the two Norwegians leapt into her and the lifeboat returned safely to the shore.

An attempt was made to salvage the steamer. Half her cargo of soda and coal was saved, but by the end of the month the effort had been abandoned. James Buckett received the R.N.L.I. Silver Medal for his bravery and leadership in the rescue. The whole village deserved one.

The Sisters - Coastguard Rescue

In June, 1873, the coastguards at Atherfield noted a schooner ashore on the ledge. She was the 120 ton *Sisters,* with a crew of 11. She had sailed onto the reef in a dense fog and was now being battered by the heavy groundswell, which broke right over the ship. The coastguards attempted to fire a rocket line at the wreck but it was too far out. Then they took the brave step of launching their own boat without waiting for the *Rescue* which was on its way. They safely brought the *Sister's* crew ashore. The schooner was a total loss, her cargo of pineapples strewn along the beach and her timbers added to the 'Atherfield Graveyard.'

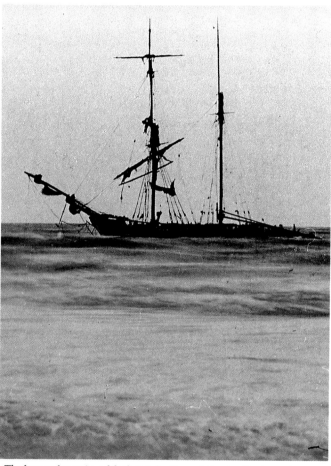

The battered remains of the brig John Douse following the dramatic rescue of her six crew in hurricane force winds. (Courtesy of the Trustees of Carisbrooke Castle Museum).

Hermose Habanero

On October 18th, 1874, the Spanish brig *Hermose Habanero* was sailing up the Channel when she was caught in a thick squall. Visibility was reduced to a few yards and the blinded vessel was driven ashore by the south-westerly wind. She came ashore at Sudmore Point at nine in the evening. The Brook boat was launched and Coxswain Hayter persuaded the Spaniards to come ashore in the lifeboat as the groundswell would have wrecked the brig's boats. The eight men were brought ashore in the early morning. The brig stood firm until the following afternoon, still under full sail. Then the mainmast finally collapsed and the rest of the ship disintegrated in half an hour. Her timbers and her cargo of sugar, rum and Mahogany were lost or scattered along the shore between Brighstone and Brook.

One of the worst winters in the Island's maritime history was that of 1877-78. In the gales that swept the Channel between October and December six ships were wrecked around the Island.

The first was the *Cloud,* a small Cowes smuggling ship with two crew. She was smashed to splinters on the rocks at Puckaster Cove on October 5th. One man was assumed drowned, the other arrested.

Desperate Rescue in Sandown Bay

One of the greatest rescues of the decade was that of the *John Douse,* in which the crew of the Bembridge lifeboat nearly sacrificed their lives.

The Falmouth brig, *John Douse,* was sailing from Rouen to Cork with a cargo of plaster when she was caught in a strong southerly gale which forced her onto the English coast. Unable to reach the Solent, Captain Tom Sanders dropped anchors in Sandown Bay and hoped the gale would drop. Instead it grew into 'a perfect hurricane,' which drove the brig so hard that she slipped her anchors and went aground at about 8 p.m.

A messenger from Sandown galloped to Bembridge to alert the lifeboat crew. At 9 p.m. the Bembridge boat, the *City of Worcester,* was ready to begin the six mile haul by road to Sandown. This was not easy, given a headwind of 70 miles an hour in exposed places, accompanied by thick driving rain. Nevertheless, it took only three hours.

When the boat was launched into the maelstrom of water that Sandown Bay had become, the *John Douse* had disappeared in the rain and darkness, her lights extinguished by the seas crashing clean over her decks, the six crew forced to take refuge in the rigging. Luckily the brig was facing the storm stern on, not broadside.

After a search lasting 1½ hours the *City of Worcester* found the wreck and closed in under the rigging. Captain Sanders dropped into the boat from a boom, and the mate dropped into the sea and was hauled aboard. Before anyone else could reach the lifeboat a tremendous sea swept her away. As she plummeted into the hollow of the huge wave her steer oar touched the bottom of the bay. A few inches lower and the lifeboat would have thrown her precious cargo into the waves, probably drowning the whole crew. Coxswain Serle 'deemed it unadvisable to approach the wreck until daylight.' A wise move. He decided to beat back to seaward of the wreck and lie off her in case of an emergency. While doing this the boat was swamped and Serle was washed overboard. The boat followed his cries, found him and hauled him back aboard.

Through the long night the lifeboatmen waited, while the wretched four men in the rigging prayed that the masts might hold, and those ashore felt their worst fears grow with every passing minute. As dawn approached, the coastguards, assuming that the *City of Worcester* was lost, launched their galley and took off the four men from the brig before the lifeboat arrived from seaward. It had been an incredible rescue. The only casualty was the brig which was a write off, her stern beaten in, the sea washing right through. Her masts had gone in two days and her remains were auctioned on November 23rd.

The following year Charles Serle retired as Bembridge Coxswain to be succeeded by Edmund Attrill, who served as Coxswain for the next 25 years.

Two Wrecks in a Day

Alpheta and *Chin Yang.* Ten days after the loss of the *John Douse,* two ships were wrecked at opposite ends of the Island on the same day, the Shoreham barque *Alpheta* and the *Chin Yang,* from St. Johns, Canada. The iron *Alpheta,* bound from Bremerhaven to Cardiff was driven onto Bembridge Ledge in a strong westerly wind and thick rain. She split her hull and began to fill with water, but without danger to the crew. Two fishing boats put eight men aboard to lend a hand, but nothing could be done and they later returned to shore with the lifeboat, along with two women and two children from the ship.

The *Chin Yang* was caught in Totland Bay while heading for the Hurst Race enroute for Southampton, with a cargo of grain. Here the wind blew from the west-north-west forcing the Canadian ship onto the rocks of Warden Ledge. Like the *Alpheta,* she bumped hard and began to fill with water, but there seemed to be no great danger to the crew.

The next day both ships were attended by tugs. A diver inspected the *Alpheta* and salvage plans were abandoned, she was broken up for scrap. On the 26th another tug, a barge and pumps came to the aid of the *Chin Yang,* which was badly damaged, full of water and stripped of her rigging. Nevertheless, she was pumped out, refloated, and towed to Yarmouth just six days later.

The final casualties of 1877 were the barge *Two Brothers,* which foundered off Ryde, and the ketch *Champion.* She was collecting stone for ship ballast from the Shingles Bank when something went badly wrong. On December 2nd she was found aground and empty, her boat was found later floating upside-down. The crew must have been trapped on the exposed bank and were swept away by the sea.

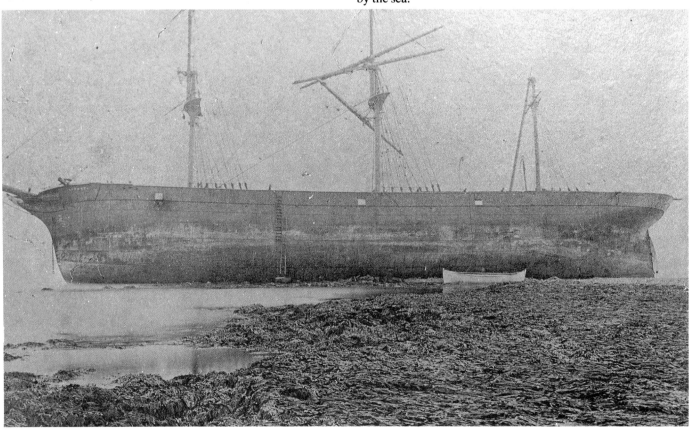

The iron barque Alpheta, stranded and later broken up on Bembridge ledge in November, 1877. (Courtesy of the Trustees of Carisbrooke Castle Museum).

The Mystery of H.M.S. Eurydice

One Sunday afternoon in March, 1878, the Bishop of Ripon and Sir John MacNiell were taking tea with Sir John Cowell in his rooms at Windsor. MacNiell was gazing out of the window when he suddenly exclaimed "Good Heavens! Why don't they close the portholes and reef the sails!" An astonished Cowell asked MacNiell what he meant, but he replied that he hardly knew, only that he had envisioned a ship coming up the Channel under full sail, her gunports open, with a great black squall descending upon her.

That same afternoon and 70 miles away, a thick driving blizzard swept out across Sandown Bay and capsized the training frigate *H.M.S. Eurydice.* Of 366 men; only two were saved.

Why is it that Captain Hare failed to take precautions against the squall? Was the whole crew drunk as one of the survivors later alleged, or was the storm hidden from view and so exceptionally violent that the ship was doomed from the moment the black cloud appeared on the northern horizon?

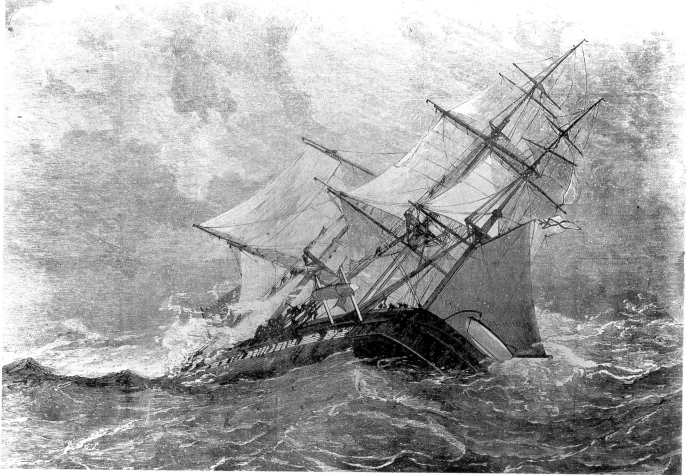

H.M.S. Eurydice capsizes in a violent snow squall off Dunnose Point, March, 1878. (From the front page of the Illustrated London News).

H.M.S. Eurydice was completed in 1843 as a 26 gun, 921 ton frigate. She was designed primarily for speed, with a sleek wooden hull and a broad expanse of sail. She aroused great admiration. "In her prime *Eurydice* was counted among the crack sailing vessels in the navy, and I have met old sailors who have shaken sorrowful heads whilst admitting that her like will never be looked upon again, who described her saucy beauty as she crowded on all plain sail and skimmed the trade crisped water like a thing of pulsing life" Built towards the close of the age of sail, the *Eurydice* was one of the finest sailing vessels ever to grace the world's oceans. Considering her refit in 1877 it seems certain that her final demise had nothing to do with the design and abilities of the ship.

By the mid-seventies the *Eurydice* and all other wooden warships were obsolete so the Admiralty ordered that she be converted into a training ship. In 1876/77 the *Eurydice* was given a complete refit at J. Whites shipyard at Cowes. On February 7th, 1877, she was recommissioned and sent to Portsmouth for a few final touches. There she came under the command of Captain Marcus Hare and an experienced cadre of officers. The 300 ordinary seamen came from a number of training ships from all over the country.

On November 13th the *Eurydice* set sail from Portsmouth for a successful three month tour of the British West Indies. In March she called at Bermuda where she picked up 35 passengers, mostly soldiers and marines from the naval dockyard.

On March 6th, 1878, the *Eurydice* set sail for Portsmouth. It was an excellent trip. She crossed the Atlantic in 16 days and with perfect navigational precision arrived off the Isle of Wight at 3 p.m. on March 22nd. Bonchurch Coastguard Station noted the ship passing at 3.30 p.m. 'moving fast under all plain sail, studding sails on fore and main, bonnets and skyscrapers.'

The ship was noted and admired by many people on the Island who were out enjoying one of the first fine days after a particularly cold and stormy winter. An artist, Ellen Sewell, sketched the ship and described it to a friend. The frigate was gliding through a 'green and purple sea' under full sail with her gunports open. The sky was blue with tall pillars of white cloud and a fresh north-westerly wind tearing the tops of the waves.

At 3.40 the ship was cutting across the bottom of Sandown Bay. There were two other ships in the area; a two man fishing boat returning from the Princessa Shoal to Shanklin, and a coal bearing

29

schooner, the *Emma,* somewhat to the south of the *Eurydice.* Between 3.40 and 3.45 Captain Jenkins of the *Emma* and Mr. Colenut, the fisherman, noted an intense black cloud growing on the northern horizon and took the necessary precautions. Colenut put in under Culver Cliff and Jenkins reefed his sails.

Sails Filled With Snow

The great squall bore down on the exposed ships in the bay, a bitterly cold 30,000 foot tower of cloud circulating at enormous speed, blackened by its weight of snow and ice. It had broken free of the main polar air mass and traversed England from the Bristol Channel leaving a trail of destruction in its wake. At 3.45 the *Eurydice* was last seen proceeding just as MacNiell saw her in Windsor, under full sail with the gunports open. Then she disappeared, enveloped by the blizzard.

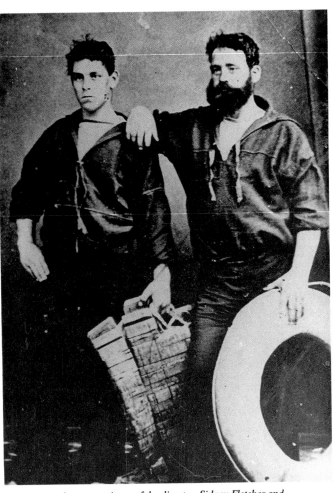

The only two survivors of the disaster, Sidney Fletcher and Benjamin Cuddiford, photographed in Ventnor shortly after the disaster. (Courtesy of the Trustees of Carisbrooke Castle Museum).

According to one of the survivors, Benjamin Cuddiford, Captain Hare was summoned to the deck just before 3.45. Realising the danger far too late, he ordered the new watch aloft to take in the upper sails and ordered all hands on deck. Even as he spoke the air before the oncoming blizzard began to back off causing the wind to swing around to the east, flattening the sails against the masts and pushing the ship off course. While Hare's orders were still being relayed and the men were just climbing the nets, the squall struck with a blast that almost knocked them off their feet. The sails slapped taught and began to fill with thick snow. A few miles away Colenut was amazed by the weather "Never have I been out in such a storm. I have never seen snow so thick." The frigate was pushed around 90 degrees to face south-east and forced over onto her starboard side. The fore and mizzen topgallant masts were torn away and the icy March sea began to gush through the open starboard ports. The second survivor, Sidney Fletcher, was below when the wind struck. By the time he reached the deck there was only enough time to grab a lifebuoy and leap overboard. Cuddiford climbed onto the port side of the hull as the ship capsized. The *Eurydice* righted herself in a final defiant gesture and then her bow was driven into the sea and plunged

towards the seabed, 11 fathoms below. Most of the crew were drowned between decks, the rest pulled off their clothes and leapt into the icy waves, most without lifebuoys. Many were sucked down with the ship. All the ship's crew were capable swimmers but the sea was at its coldest after the long winter months, little above freezing. The surface of the sea was now a chaos of leaping waves blanketed under a thick deluge of snow. Despite their youth and strength the majority of the survivors were soon paralysed by the cold and sank beneath the angry waves. For the few survivors lucky enough to have lifebuoys to hold up their chilled bodies, it was now a question of staying alive until the squall passed, a supreme battle of will and physical endurance. The blizzard continued for 45 minutes.

At 4.30 it ceased as suddenly as it had begun, and the sun shone down on an empty sea where the frigate had been. Captain Jenkins of the *Emma* resumed his journey but was soon horrified to see the topmost sails of the *Eurydice* flapping above the water. He then saw some bodies and tacked his ship to reach them. The schooner's boat picked up five men at about 5 p.m. One was dead on arrival at the ship and two more by the time the *Emma* reached Ventnor. The two survivors were taken to Ventnor Cottage Hospital where they recovered.

The site of the tragedy was soon busy with naval vessels and tugs, and salvage work began almost immediately. The frigate was raised soon after and beached on Bembridge Ledge, looking like a beached whale. She was never recommissioned. Her bell now hangs in St. Paul's Church, Shanklin.

The Eurydice's Ghost

Soon after the disaster people using the bay began telling eerie tales of a phantom three masted ship which vanished if it was approached. Freak reflections of light on the mist were blamed but these hardly explain the sighting by Commander F. Lipscomb and members of his crew in the 1930's. Their submarine was obliged to take evasive action to avoid striking a full rigged ship, only to see it disappear. When Lipscomb came to the Island to enquire of the strange sighting, he was told that he had seen the *Eurydice.*

The Unresolved Mystery

Both the Isle of Wight Coroner and the Court Martial 'attached no blame whatever to the captain, officers and men of the ship' but neither solved the central mystery of why the crew did not take action to save the ship before it was too late.

One solution is offered by geography. At the time when the squall was first seen, the *Eurydice* was still rounding Dunnose Point so that the black cloud was partly hidden from view by the 800 foot high mass of St. Boniface Down.

A far more cynical explanation was offered by Sidney Fletcher who took a minor part in the two trials. Years later he told his family that the truth was that the whole crew had been drinking for hours and were 'as high as kites, officers and men,' and didn't know what they were doing, many being unconscious in their hammocks. This is passed down hearsay but it does have a ring of truth. The ship's company had a lot to celebrate that sunny afternoon. It was their last day together after a successful three month cruise and they were looking forward to their homecoming. Captain Hare no doubt relaxed the ship's rigid discipline but it is unlikely that officers of his calibre were 'high as kites.' What is more likely is that a combination of too much rum and an atmosphere of casual over-confidence; like that aboard the *Royal George* a century before; laid the ship wide open to an unexpected but totally avoidable disaster.

Three Spectacular Shipwrecks: 1879-1881

The two years between January, 1879 and January, 1881 provided a particularly busy time for the sea rescue services on the Island. Three of the most dramatic wrecks of the century occurred along with a good number of other casualties. These were the three barques *Schiehallion*, the *Alpheus Marshall* and the *Atlas*.

Thanks to the Board of Trade wreck inquiry held on the Captain and Mate of the fine 600 ton barque *Schiehallion*, we are furnished with most of the details of the ship's final hours. Two lives and all the cargo was lost with the ship and it seems that her Captain, John Levack, must take much of the blame.

The *Schiehallion* left Auckland, New Zealand, in September, 1878, with 16 crew, 13 passengers and about 700 tons of Rosnum gum. She was a good ship, just ten years old and rated 'A1' by Lloyds Shipping. Captain Levack was a part owner of the vessel. He had been at sea for 32 years, commanded ships for 17, and had never had an accident.

Careless Navigation

On January 11th 1879, Levack wandered on deck just as the lights of the Isles de Vierge (off Brittany) were falling below the horizon. From them he guessed his position and set a course for mid channel. The barque battled with headwinds until 2 a.m. and was then becalmed for three and a half hours. How Levack knew his position after that is anyone's guess but he set a course the next morning that he expected would take the ship a few miles south of St. Catherine's. He was remarkably accurate but he didn't realise that while his ship had been becalmed it had drifted four miles north in 'Rennels Current.'

On the early morning of the 13th the *Schiehallion* was sailing directly towards St. Catherine's. At 4 a.m. Levack retired below telling the Mate, James Lyall, to watch out for the lighthouse. Lyall was himself a qualified master but he lacked both the initiative to check his position and his Captain's natural instinct. He had two lookouts forward to cope with the fog which lay in thick banks bordered by clear areas of open sea. The keeper at St. Catherine's was looking at six miles of clear seascape. The solemn drone of the foghorn did not sound until 7 a.m.

At 5.15 the *Schiehallion* approached a high dense bank of fog that completely hid the Island's coast. A quarter of an hour later the doomed ship cracked her keel on the submerged boulders of Rocken End.

A Suicidal Proposition

Levack was on deck in a matter of seconds and ordered the sails to be furled and distress rockets to be fired, but there was nothing else he could do. The big groundswell and the steep rocky shore made landing with the ship's three boats a suicidal proposition. However, the 29 people aboard had to get off the ship as the

groundswell was pushing her hard against the rocks causing her to crack and split and fill with water. She slid down deeper and settled onto her starboard side. The ship's only hope lay with the Niton Life Saving Apparatus, manned by a company of coastguards, but the ship had come ashore at a point where the land rises 600 feet in a chaotic series of sandstone cliffs and ledges, over and down which the Niton men had to manhandle the rocket, tripod, ropes and accessories. It was a race against time and the people on the sinking barque felt they were losing, as they clung to the portside railings and watched the sea pounding the exposed deck. In desperation the ship's cook offered to swim through the rock-strewn surf with a rope tied around his middle. To the cheers of all aboard he was pulled out of the sea and the rope secured. One by one people aboard came ashore, hand over hand, drenched and frozen by the waves. Half way across, the Second Mate lost his grip and disappeared into the surf.

By now the rocket apparatus had been set up and fired and soon both lines were busy bringing the shivering survivors ashore. It was not a moment too soon. One boy was swept from the port rail and drowned among the rocks. Levack stuck to his ship like a good captain, being the last but one ashore.

The crew and passengers saved nothing from the *Schiehallion*. She rapidly broke up in the swell and the fast tidal currents and was widely scattered along the southern coast. As late as 1941 one might still find bits of Rosnum gum from her cargo as far away as Luccombe Beach.

Both Levack and Lyall were arraigned before a wreck inquiry at Westminster in February. Lyall was acquitted but the Wreck Commissioner said that Levack had disregarded the primary duty of 'determining accurately his position.' His Master's licence was suspended for six months.

The Alpheus Marshall

Less than a month after the loss of the *Schiehallion*, on February 9th, 1879, the villagers of Brighstone gathered for Divine Service in St. Mary's Church. It was a foul night. Above the howling of the wind and the distant thunder along the beach, the sound of the lifeboat cannon broke the atmosphere. The service was immediately abandoned, and congregation, vicar and choir filed out into the gathering darkness to run down to the lifeboat house at Grange Chine. The call was for the New York barque *Alpheus Marshall*, which had been sailing from Nova Scotia to London with

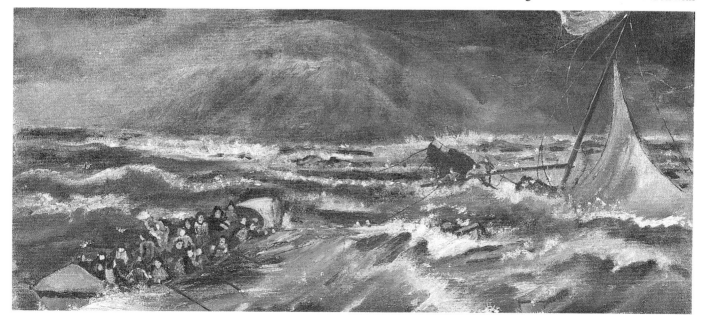

"The Wreck of the Alpheus Marshall" by Felicity Edwards.

a general cargo and 14 crew. She was rudely interrupted by storm force winds blowing up-Channel. The barque was driven almost helplessly onto the waiting rocks of the Atherfield Ledge. She struck hard and was pushed around by the swell so that her bow pointed into the storm. Enormous seas buried the ship under a blanket of spray and spume. Her hull was shattered against the unyielding rocks and soon settled under the pounding waves. When the Brighstone boat *Rescue* finally reached the scene after an epic launch and a long struggle against the wind, only the three masts and the starboard side of the poop still showed above the water.

Shattered on the Rocks

Coxswain James Buckett knew he couldn't get too close for fear of being cast up on the rocks. Instead the *Rescue* carefully approached from seaward and connected a rope to the spanker boom. One by one the American crew fought their way through the storm-tossed seas to the lifeboat. Back on board the hatch covers exploded under the enormous pressures and the ship began to come apart. The lifeboat was badly overloaded and was being continually swamped by the huge seas breaking across the Ledge. When all 14 men were aboard, Buckett took the boat straight into the shore, but he found that the waves were breaking right up against the cliffs. There was no beach to land on and the boats' helpers could not hook the *Rescue's* bow and pull her in. (Just being hit by one of those waves can knock one unconscious, and the helpers had been forced up the cliff). Still, Buckett had no choice.

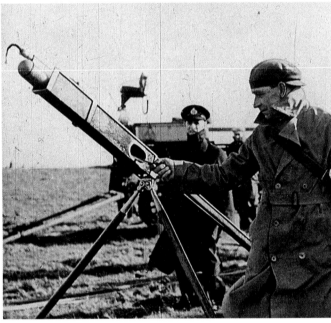

The Boxer Rocket about to be fired.

The lifeboat struck the steeply shelving shore and swung broadside onto the beach. The next big breaker crashed down on the boat washing out all 27 men, half of them without lifejackets. Risking all, the helpers rushed into the surf to pull them towards the cliff. A few were sucked back into deep water by the powerful 'backsend,' but were returned by the next rush of the sea. Somehow all 27 men were dragged from the cold greedy grip of that terrible storm. Most were injured but all were alive.

Coxswain James Buckett decided that his time had come to retire. He was 74 and had been the Brighstone Coxswain for nearly 20 years. His son Captain Buckett recalled of him: "He saved 280 lives altogether . . . and from being an outlaw became a public favourite on whose birthday the Church bells used to be rung." His place was filled by the Second Coxswain, Moses Munt.

When the *Alpheus Marshall* broke up she left a kind legacy for the people who had rescued her crew as 14 lbs. tins of beef and tinned prawns and tomatoes washed up in the surf. Despite the half-hearted efforts of the coastguards most of this flotsam ended up being hidden in smuggler's stashes. Mr. W. Green of Brighstone recalled that the tomatoes provided something of a mystery. "We did not know they were 'til we were told. But the whole cargo was much appreciated. When I came home for weekends my mother used to ask me to get another tin of beef. It was a Godsend to many a poor family."

Several other ships wrecked, grounded or foundered at this time but the next spectacular loss was the 554 ton Austrian barque *Atlas*. She was carrying maize from New York to Papenburg in Germany when she was swept off course by a fresh south-westerly gale and a series of sudden squalls.

The Desperate Plight of the Atlas

At 7 a.m. on November 25th, 1880, she was driven onto the now infamous rocks of Atherfield Ledge. The coastguards quickly alerted the lifeboat station at Brighstone and the brand new boat *The Worcester Cadet* was brought down Grange Chine to the sea. The new coxswain, Moses Munt, was a great seaman and leader but that day was to prove too much for him and his crew. The launch was successful but the journey to the crazed white waters of the Ledge was a long bitter struggle in the face of direct headwinds. Munt found that he could make no progress towards the ailing wreck. As Lloyds Lists unkindly reported: "The lifeboat, mismanaged, drifted to leeward and could not make weather way against the tide and was quite useless." The struggle to make headway pushed the crew beyond the limits of exhaustion and they had to return to station. There two of the men were almost carried out of the boat. The Atherfield coastguards tried next. Five lifesaving rockets were fired but each was thrown aside by the gale. They also launched their own boat into that terrible sea but it was soon swamped and several of the coastguards washed out of her. It was as much as they could manage to save themselves and get back to the beach alive.

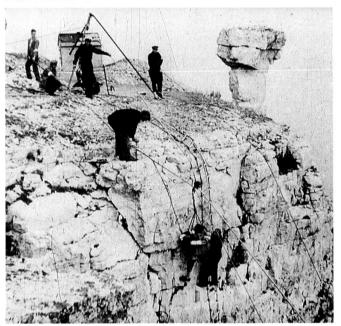

The Breeches Buoy in operation. Note the tripod and cliff ladder.

Things were getting desperate aboard the *Atlas*. Her back was broken and great seas were sweeping her decks. Her torn sails testified to the violence of the gusting wind. Her maintopmast was carried away and it was apparent to all that the crew, who were sheltering in the rigging, had little time left to get off the ship alive.

Seeing that the people ashore could do nothing, one of the crew came down to the deck and tied a tub to a long piece of rope and threw it over the side. As he had hoped, the tub washed towards the shore but it caught on some rocks before reaching the beach. It seemed that the attempt had failed until coastguardman Jimmy Fairweather "plunged into the surf and after a struggle secured the tub and brought it to land amid the cheers of the spectators." The rope was tied to a hawser and hauled back to the ship by its crew. Under the able direction of Captain Vidulich the hawser was attached to the mainmast and a bosun's chair hoisted out to the ship. One by one the shipwrecked men were hauled across the angry surf, many being injured as they were thrown about by the leaping waves. Vidulich was the last man ashore. It had been a brilliant rescue.

There was never much chance of saving the ship or its cargo. The ship quickly commenced to break up, the shore being strewn with maize and wreckage of all descriptions. The *Atlas* completely disappeared in two days and the crew lost all their belongings. The ugly black rocks of Atherfield had claimed yet another victim.

Steamers on the Rocks 1881-1886

Over a period of five years, no less than six steamers ploughed into the western shores of the Island. These losses were mainly due to fog, aided by careless navigation. These ships brought great benefit to the 'Back of the Wight' in the form of salvage work, as well as the usual theft of wreck.

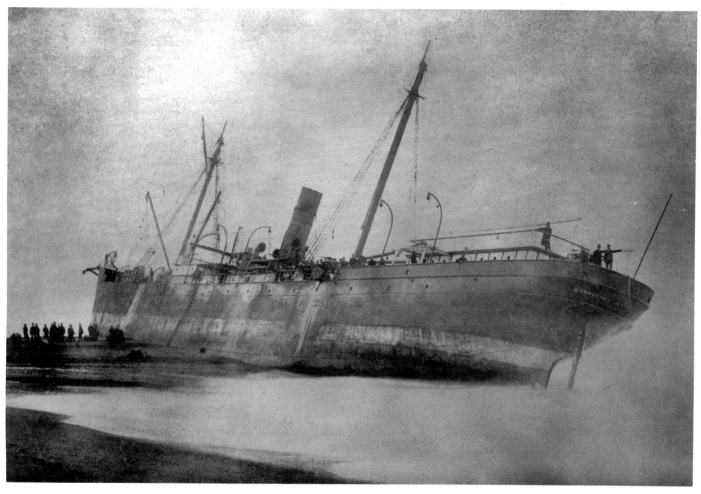

The S.S. Cormorant, stranded close to Whale Chine in Chale Bay, December 21st, 1886.

S.S. Claremont

Typical of these casualties was the Newcastle steamer *Claremont* which came ashore at Whale Chine on January 27th, 1881. She was just ten years old and weighed 1,023 tons gross. She was on her way to Middlesbrough with a cargo of iron and copper ore and 20 crew under the command of Captain Bainbridge. He noted Portland at 11 a.m. but he did not take any bearings, which was a mistake, as the cold mist thickened into a particularly dense fog as the afternoon progressed. Bainbridge casually posted a lookout in the foc'sle, but did not reduce speed and failed to check the depth with the lead. *Claremont* ploughed on at ten knots, well off course, thanks to a strong spring flood tide, and with a lookout who sometimes could not see more than 12 feet ahead.

Blissfully unaware of the danger, Bainbridge went below at 5 p.m. Half an hour later *Claremont's* bow smashed onto the steeply sloping beach of Chale Bay. Bainbridge rushed to the bridge and ordered the engines full astern. The 99 horse-power engines thundered away until the engineer reported that the boilers were coming apart, and they were then shut down. One seaman rowed off to get help, eventually arriving at Ventnor; while the rest abandoned the ship into two larger boats, one under Bainbridge, and one under the Mate. The ship was groaning loudly and the heavy groundswell meant that the crew could not land their boats straight onto the beach. When *Claremont's* iron back broke, the two boats set off into the dense fog and soon lost one another.

Back on land Coxswain Moses Munt had heard the *Claremont's* siren and alerted the crew of the *Worcester Cadet* which commenced a long search in the freezing fog. They found the Mate's boat with five men aboard, and brought them to shore at 3.40 a.m. The Captain's luck with navigation had not improved.

The following morning found him and the remaining 13 crew drifting off Luccombe. Fortunately they were picked up by the tug *Victoria* which was on her way to salvage the *Claremont*. This proved to be impossible, as her hull was broken and the cargo was washing away.

The Board of Trade enquiry found Bainbridge responsible for the loss and suspended his licence for six months.

S.S. Essen

The following month the German steamer *Essen*, also loaded with Spanish iron ore came ashore early one morning at Rocken End. It was high tide, and when it ebbed Captain Jurgensen and his crew simply walked ashore. The *Essen* was a total wreck.

S.S. Wheatfield

The 1,200 ton steamer *Wheatfield* beached at Blackgang on New Year's Eve, 1882. She had been bound from Lieth to New York with a general cargo when she broke down in the Channel and was driven ashore. The crew abandoned ship immediately as she had begun to break up. They came ashore at the foot of the Chine where luckily some of the Wheeler family caught the boats and pulled them in to safety. Meanwhile the steamer's welcome cargo of meat and flour was beginning to wash ashore. "Here was a chance too good to be missed," recalled Fred Mew, "and soon bags of flour and tins of beef were climbing the cliff in all directions. The police and coastguards had a busy time, while occasionally the men in blue could be seen briskly setting off with a tin of beef to be put in some hiding place till the coast was clear". The *Wheatfield* was well remembered as the 'Flour Ship.' She helped to "fill many larders and empty tummies!"

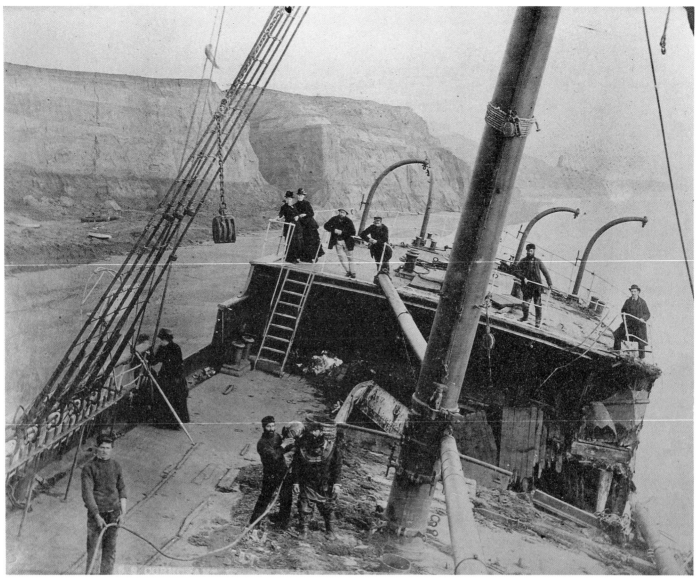

The deck of the Cormorant during salvage operations. Note the diver and the gash torn into the ship by another vessel which rammed the Cormorant in the fog. Her white figurehead lies close to the stairway.

S.S. Castle Craig

On December 14th, 1883, the *Castle Craig* was steaming up the Channel from Odessa, in the Black Sea, loaded with Russian grain, oil and feathers. When she entered into a dense mass of fog she lost her bearings and drove onto Brook Ledge. The crew of the *George and Anne* were summoned at the unsocial hour of 4 a.m. and launched into the heavy freezing seas. The R.N.L.I. Journal reports that "much difficulty and danger was incurred in laying near to the vessel so as to take the crew off, but eventually this was safely accomplished." In two trips the lifeboat brought ashore all 31 of the crew.

The Duke of Westminster

The biggest wreck yet seen on the Island was the four masted 4,426 ton *Duke of Westminster*. She came ashore on the rocks of Atherfield on January 3rd, 1884. As she was a new steel built ship she was able to withstand the winter weather during the weeks of salvage work and thus became one of the first ships to escape the "dreaded Atherfield Ledge."

The big screw steamer came ashore thanks to faulty navigation and the failure of her master Captain Cox to check his depth. She was steaming from Australia to London with a general cargo and 20 passengers. As she was both a sailing ship and a steamer she had 102 crew, mostly 'Lascars,' low paid Asiatic sailors. When she entered the Channel the big ship lost sight of land in a thick fog, and shifted course 7 degrees north thanks to faulty bearings taken off Portland. As a result she ploughed onto the outer rocks of Atherfield Ledge at full speed at just before six on the evening of January 3rd.

As soon as he realised the situation Captain Cox ordered the engines full astern. For a few minutes the 350 horse power engines screwed the sea astern into a white boiling tumult, but the big steamer was out of luck. As often happens there was a big swell running and as the ship's stern rose and fell, her propellor blades were sheared off on the rocks below. Cox had another idea. A boat was lowered and dropped two kedge anchors astern. Then the ship's great steam winches began to haul in the thick anchor chains, dragging the steamer safely off the reef into five fathoms of water. However, the slack allowed the anchors to come free. Another anchor was dropped to steady the ship's crumpled bows, but the stern swung round on the swell, and with ponderous grace she grounded heavily on the ledge denting her plates and cracking her sternpost. The huge ship was now completely crippled.

The Brighstone boat, *Worcester Cadet,* arrived that night and took off the passengers. Tugs soon arrived to assist the vessel but they could not budge her, and as the weather worsened over the next few days the whole crew had to be evacuated; the last 53 men being landed at Atherfield in three trips by the *Worcester Cadet* on January 5th.

After a battering that would have destroyed any iron ship in that position, the stranded steamer was unloaded of her cargo by teams of shore hands. The perishable cargo of oranges and coconuts was jettisoned, a welcome bonus to those on shore. Once empty, after weeks of work, the badly damaged ship was at last pulled free of the ledge and towed to London for repairs. Captain Cox had his Master's licence taken away for six months after a Board of Trade Inquiry.

S.S. Cormorant

The Scottish steamer *Cormorant* left New Orleans for Bremen on November 27th, 1886 with a cargo of raw cotton. She had a crew of 33 under Captain James Lowe, and weighed 2,255 tons gross. Lowe was an experienced master, he had served the Bird Line for 21 years, and commanded ships for 11.

As the ship steamed up the Channel on the night of December 20th, she entered a dense fog. Through the bitterly cold night the fog cut down visibility to only 50 yards. Twice Lowe altered course to the north to get a bearing from the land, but he did not reduce speed and he did not try casting a lead. At 6.50 a.m. he went to the Chart Room to work out his position. He calculated that the ship was seven or eight miles S. S.W. of St. Catherine's. Reassured, he returned to the deck to be confronted by a cliff 50 yards ahead. "Hard to port" he yelled, but the ship was done for. With all the momentum of over 2,000 tons being pushed by 230 horse-power engines the *Cormorant's* bow ploughed into a soft bed of shingle and clay. For an hour the engines thundered full astern with no effect. Dawn found the ship high on the beach close to Whale Chine. She had come ashore at high water which made getting her off that much more difficult.

"Hurrah! She's ours!"

That day a tug arrived, and watched by a big crowd on the cliff-top, she commenced to tow the stranded steamer off. The chances for it were good, as Fred Mew recalled "The wind was now south, with a heavy swell running, an ideal time to float her, as a south wind sends more water into the bay, and when the big swells came, she was almost afloat." Just as the iron hull began to slip back into her natural element, the hawser parted, and pushed by the southern swell, her stern swung broadside onto the beach. On the cliff-top some of the people flung their caps into the air shouting "Hurrah! She's ours!" They knew the ship could not be saved, and this would mean plenty of work.

However, the ships crew and the salvors had not given up yet. Two more tugs arrived with barges, and the crew began to jettison the cargo to lighten the ship. "This was promptly rolled up under the cliff by those ashore, this being the commencement of a good cotton harvest."

Now the weather stepped in to seal the fate of the ship. The wind increased to gale force making it impossible for the barges to get close to her, and later, blowing in seas that crashed clean over the vessel. As the deck was leaning towards the sea this meant that the crew had to abandon the vessel at 3 p.m. The storm continued for two days.

By midday of the 23rd Lloyds reported that the ship was lying with a 35 degree angle to the sea, her rudder broken, the ruptured iron hull filling with the tide, and her deck fittings and boats broken off and strewn along the beach towards Rocken End.

Salvage Work

The following day gangs of men were hired from around the Island to unload the cotton bales. The bales were lowered to the beach with the ship's derricks and then dragged up the cliff by teams of horses. They were stacked into massive piles and then rumbled off on carts to Newport. All the local carters and their horses were employed. Naturally some of the cotton was stolen. As it was wet and weighed more, it could not be checked. Once the wreck was emptied, it was sold and broken up, providing work for several years. Never has a wreck brought such material benefit to the poor of the 'Back of the Wight.'

Shortly after the salvage began, an extraordinary thing happened. Arriving for work the salvors found a huge gash in the wreck's side, and a strange figurehead lying on the deck. When the mist cleared a ship was seen anchored in the bay, her bows badly damaged. She had rammed the *Cormorant* during the night and then managed to escape.

The Board of Trade inquiry into the loss of the *Cormorant* found Lowe guilty of "wrongful acts and defaults" and suspended his licence for six months.

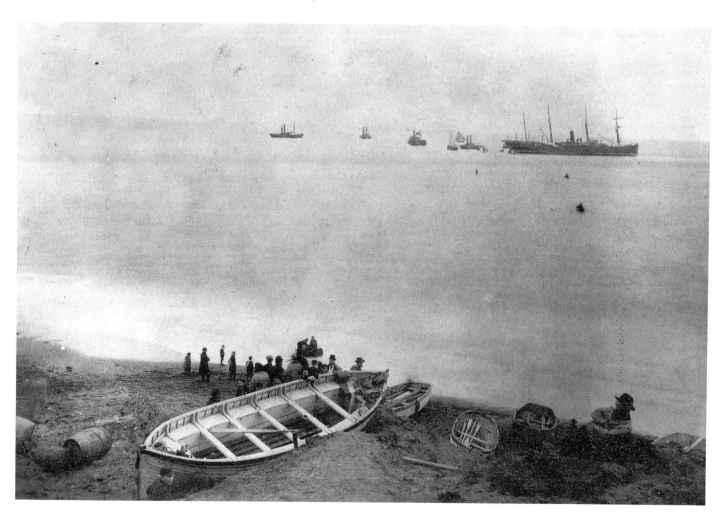

The 4,426 ton Duke of Westminster aground on Atherfield Ledge and undergoing salvage operations, January, 1884. Note the ship's lifeboat and the local fishing boats in the foreground.

The Sirenia Disaster

On March the 9th and 10th, 1888, the crews of the Brighstone and Brook lifeboats made four extraordinary attempts to rescue the 31 people trapped aboard the full rigged *Sirenia*. They pitted their strength and skills against conditions so extreme that the launch of the boats was almost impossible, let alone the rescue. They were tested up to and beyond the limits of physical endurance. In saving all but two of the ship's company in an epic rescue, both boats Second Coxswains were drowned, along with Moses Munt, the Brighstone Coxswain, and both crews were put out of action.

"On the morning of March 9th, 1888, there was a dense fog and a surprisingly heavy sea," wrote Lord Mottistone in his book 'Launch.' "It often happens on our coast, that when a fog comes on without a breath of wind, great rollers come tumbling in; first with a boom like distant thunder as occasional waves break on the outer ledges; then with a loud continuous roar, as the waves from the Atlantic increase in size so that each one breaks on the outer ledge, and then, pressed forward by its follower, gathers impetus to hurl itself on the shore. Meanwhile there is still the uncanny absence of wind to account for this great disturbance of the sea. So it was when the *Sirenia* struck on Atherfield Ledge." "I was on a job, building a barn for my father," recalls Mr. Buckett, a member of the Brighstone lifeboat crew. "The fog was very thick, and the sea was making that noise that I suppose it was in the heads of all of us that we hoped the lifeboat would not be wanted."

That afternoon young Harry Cotton was walking along the Atherfield shore towards Chale. Hearing a noise and looking towards the fogbound ocean, he saw a great white cloud billowing above the ledge. He realised that it was a big ship that had run aground under full sail. He climbed the cliff and ran breathless to his father's cottage. Rufus Cotton jumped to his feet at the news and ran off to warn the rest of the Brighstone crew.

The stranded ship, the *Sirenia*, of Glasgow, was a big three-masted full rigged ship with a strong iron and steel hull. She weighed 1,588 tons and carried 31 people including Captain MacIntyre, his wife, three children, their woman servant and 25 crew. She was just completing the long voyage from San Francisco via Cape Horn, with a cargo of wheat bound for Dunkirk.

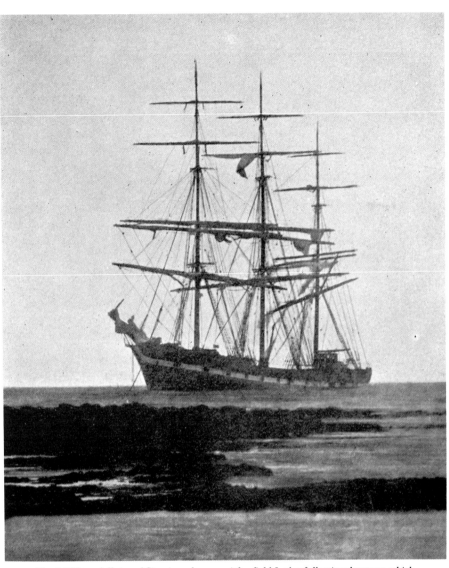

The 1,588 ton full rigged Sirenia, ashore on Atherfield Ledge following the storm which claimed the lives of two of her crew and three local lifeboatmen.
(Courtesy of the I.W. County Press).

Like many others she had drifted off course in the fog on the incoming tide, until she ran heavily aground on an outer reef of 'the dreaded Atherfield Ledge.' MacIntyre had no idea of the danger that his ship was in. When a pilot lugger, the *Renown*, from Deal, sailed right around his ship and offered to take off everyone aboard, he declined the offer saying he hoped to get off with the tide.

At 4 o'clock the Brighstone lifeboat cannon roared above the continuous thunder of the sea. Here there was no complacency.

Perilous Launch Into Icy Seas

Buckett ran down to take his place at the oars behind the bowman. "I had been out in the boat often before in big storms of wind, but I never saw such a big sea breaking on the beach as then. But Munt, our coxswain, was a wonderful man. He chose the right way and we got off in fine style." There was still no wind so the crew had to heave their way down the coast to Atherfield Ledge with the ten sturdy oars, climbing a succession of long grey mountainous seas. On arrival at the stricken ship the lifeboatmen were thrown a line so that they could hang onto the bow, but a big sea snapped the hawser and drove the lifeboat half the distance back to the shore.

The crew fought their way back to the ship and tied up again with a thicker line. For an hour the Brighstone men were repeatedly soaked by a deluge of icy water as each swell broke over the lifeboat's bow. One by one, the children and the two women were carefully lowered along the rope. The smallest was a baby, stowed in a whicker laundry basket. Coxswain Munt became worried about the children being washed out of the boat and knew that landing it at high tide would be bad enough without a full load of men aboard. MacIntyre agreed and told him to come back for the crew at low water.

"It was a long pull back again for there was no wind to help us and we constantly had to turn head to sea to meet the breaking waves." The lifeboat reached the Atherfield shore and was safely beached at 6.30. While the crew had been battling with the seas, the launchers had brought the boat's carriage down to the cliff at Atherfield and had somehow lowered it on ropes over the edge, at least 75 feet above the roaring sea. Atherfield cliff face is not sheer, it is made of soft black soil that is deeply terraced and slipped. Getting the carriage to the shore intact was a remarkable achievement. A few of the lifeboatmen went home to change, the rest lived too far away and had to stand and shiver and wait.

Six miles away the Brook cannon sounded and her crew pulled out the *William Slaney Lewis*. After watching the huge seas that were sweeping the bay, Coxswain John Hayter decided that it would be suicidal to launch from the bottom of the chine, and the carriage was wheeled onto the Military coast road and pulled to Brighstone. When the *William Slaney Lewis* was propelled from her carriage at Grange Chine she was lifted up by the sea and thrown on her side. Two men were injured and some oars broken. The hour-long process of restoring the boat to her carriage having been accomplished, she was hauled back up the road to the overgrown and steep Chilton Chine. Some cut away the undergrowth while the others manhandled the heavy boat and carriage down to the sea, often slipping on the wet clay. At last the boat was lined up to the waves and at Hayter's yell: "Launch!" the boat shot into the sea and successfully pulled out into deep water.

Back at Atherfield, the Brighstone crew felt the first southerly airs brush their hardened faces. "First just a gust or two from the south, then a real sou-wester; so we knew there was no time to lose in getting back to the ship by low water."

The Brighstone Boat Capsized

"Munt guessed right again and we made a fine launch. This time we could set sail." As the *Worcester Cadet* closed on the wreck she was repeatedly swamped. The waves were bigger than ever. MacIntyre shouted down to Munt that he had 13 men ready to be taken off. "We threw the grapnel into the fore-rigging and it held. Then we drifted so that the boat was alongside. Sometimes our boat was level with the rail, the next moment she was twenty feet below. In spite of all our efforts to fend her off, we hit her three times with such force that I thought our boat must be broken to bits. I think we broke at least ten oars in trying to get the boat alongside. But the thirteen men managed to jump in, or slide down a rope."

The boat being full, Munt now had to decide the exact time for casting off. As Buckett relayed Munt's shouted order to the bowman he turned and saw "a great wave in the dim light coming at us. It was worse than any of the others, like a mountain of black water, with a fringe of white on top. It took several blows of the bowman's axe to sever the thick rope, so the boat swung free just in time to be swept away by this huge racing sea. Up went the bow, higher and higher, while I held onto the thwart. I could see Munt and the thirteen men tumbling onto him just straight below me." Completely out of control the boat was driven towards the shore "at a terrific rate." When the wave finally passed beneath, it left the lifeboat bobbing broadside onto the next wave which struck almost immediately "with a crash like thunder," capsizing the boat and throwing its occupants into the sea. In a moment or two the boat righted herself with a jerk. 22 of the 26 men managed to regain her, but both Moses Munt and Thomas Cotton, the Second Coxswain, along with two of the rescued mariners were missing. With only four oars left it was hopeless trying to find them. "We shouted and burnt a flare, but in that great sea it's no wonder that we couldn't see them." The crew then steered the boat to shore where it was dragged safely onto the beach by the eager crowd of onlookers.

The crew of the *Worcester Cadet* was finished. Both her officers were dead and eight more men were sent home, including Buckett. "Most of us were pretty well knocked out by broken ribs, exhaustion and cold." For the time being the only hope for the men of the *Sirenia* lay with the arrival of the *William Slaney Lewis*.

Brook Boat Swamped

The Brook boat was now in sight of the stricken *Sirenia*. Coxswain John Hayter had already sailed his boat six miles "through a veritable Hell of waters" and was just 300 yards from the wreck when he saw a monstrous wave riding up out of the darkness. The lifeboat was nearly thrown onto her side, and three of her crew, the Second Coxswain Reuben Cooper, and the two Jacobs brothers were swept away by the sea. Luckily the Jacobs were holding onto ropes and when the boat recovered they were hauled gasping back aboard. The Brook men then set off in the direction of Coopers' cries for help, which were also clearly heard aboard the *Sirenia* as he was dragged past in the current. As the lifeboat neared the *Sirenia* Hayter yelled to MacIntyre that he could take his men off. MacIntyre insisted that the lifeboat continue the search for Cooper and fired flares to aid their search. Their sinking blue glare reflected from the raging waters, showed

the tattered wreck breaking each massive wave, and the little lifeboat bucking across the venomous ledge in the search for Cooper's frozen body.

The Brook Boat Beaten Again

The *William Slaney Lewis* rowed right across the ledge, then a maelstrom of leaping icy waves. The crew were "pounded and drenched by the huge breakers." Once clear of these terrible waters, with no hope now of finding Cooper alive, and lacking the energy to beat back to the wreck, Hayter was obliged to drop anchor and await the light of dawn. Through the remainder of that fierce night the Brook men sat and shuddered with the cold. They had all been drenched in the freezing March seas. As they sat and bandaged their blistered hands they had plenty of time to consider the closeness of death, and they must have realised that if they attempted to row back to the wreck they were all very likely to die.

As the blackened sky softened to a windswept grey, the anchor of the *William Slaney Lewis* was raised and the thick oars creaked in their rowlocks as the tired cold muscles of the Brook men began to pull the lifeboat back towards the distant masts of the *Sirenia*. The weather had not improved. The ledge remained a chaos of driving white breakers which beat and smashed over the lifeboat as it struggled slowly forward. The people ashore were horrified. They began to yell and shout into the wind and made frantic signals to Hayter to give up the attempt. Hayter noted the *Worcester Cadet* standing ready for launching on its carriage. After a long struggle the strength of the oarsmen began to give out. Several of the oars were smashed and there were no more spares. In the words of the R.N.L.I. Inquiry "the immediate return to station was the only course open to the coxswain." Hayter raised sail and made for Brook. When they arrived back it was noted that the boat had been out for fifteen hours.

The Final Effort

Attention now returned to the *Worcester Cadet*, and the beach at Atherfield, where an agitated crowd was choosing a new crew They could not wait for the weather to improve. The *Sirenia* was in a pitiful condition. The gnarled reefs had torn through her iron hull which was full of water and breaking in half. The wet cargo of wheat had begun to swell, forcing up the decks which were splintered and shattered. The remaining 13 men were crowded onto the forecastle where they had been confined for twenty hours.

Back on shore the new crew was taking shape. Rufus Cotton, the man who had raised the alarm the day before, and one of the three crewmen capable of making a third attempt to reach the shipwreck, was chosen as the coxswain. The other two were David Cotton and Frank Salter. Salter was only 19 and some tried to dissuade him. "Let me have a drink of tea and I can manage," he calmly replied. Among the new men were Edmund Attrill, the coxswain of the Bembridge boat. He had set off from Bembridge and had walked fifteen miles across the galeswept Island, clad in his heavy seaboots, to offer his services at the oars. Two others came from Sandown and one from Ventnor. Walter White, later the Atherfield coxswain, Fred Bastiani, a notorious local smuggler, John Cotton, Percy Wheeler and Charles Orchard completed the crew.

At noon the *Worcester Cadet* was launched for the third time into the terrible sea and slowly battled to the great wreck on the ledge. The remaining 13 men were taken off one by one and the lifeboat made her way safely home to the hoarse cheers of the crowd on the beach just two hours later. The lifeboat men had finally triumphed over the tempest.

As is the procedure, the Royal National Lifeboat Institution held an inquiry into the disaster which analysed the decisions of the two coxswains. The findings exonerated both Munt and Hayter. It congratulated everyone concerned with the rescue, particularly noting the courage of the crews who refused to admit defeat even under the most hopeless circumstances.

John Hayter, Rufus Cotton, David Cotton and Frank Salter received Silver Medals for their part in the rescue. The Institution gave £300 to the fund set up for the families of the deceased, and provided the fine gravestones that still stand in St. Mary's churchyard at Brighstone. The public response to the *Sirenia* disaster was magnificent. £1,200 was raised on the Island and plans were immediately made to set up a new station to watch over the Atherfield Ledge, which was opened just three and a half years later.

The Doomed Voyage of the Irex

After a doomed maiden voyage, the full rigged *Irex* came ashore at the Needles on January 25th, 1890. She was the biggest sailing ship ever to become a total wreck on the Island's shores. 29 lives were saved thanks to a record breaking rocket launch and the gallantry of local coastguards, soldiers and local people. This is a tale of extraordinary bravery in the face of terrifying circumstances.

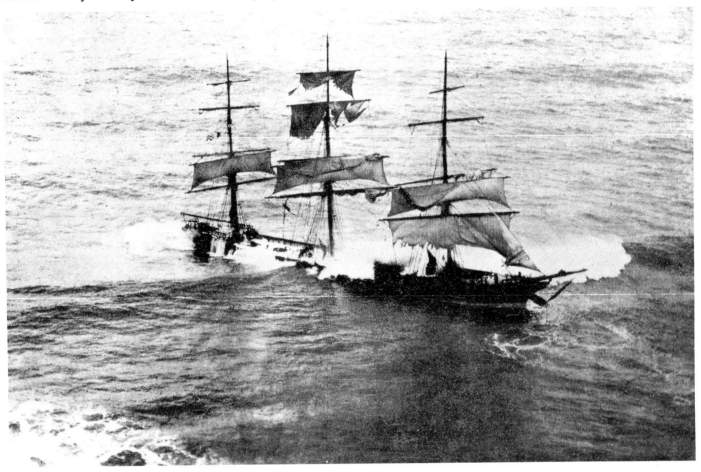

The full rigged ship Irex aground in Scratchells Bay following the rescue of her crew by rocket apparatus.

On December 10th, 1889, the bustling waters of the Clyde were graced with a majestic sight as the brand new 2,347 ton *Irex* was towed from Greenock to the Irish Sea, bound for Rio de Janeiro. The 302 feet of her sleek steel hull shone with new paint. Her three freshly varnished masts reached 200 feet into the sky. Beneath the wide hatches was carefully stowed over 3,500 tons of iron and earthenware pipes, pig iron and pots. She carried 34 crew, her experienced master, Captain Hutton, three other officers, 23 men and seven boys. Later, two stowaways were added to the crew.

The ship's troubles began almost as soon as she set sail. A violent south-westerly gale shifted the heavy cargo, forcing Hutton to run her back to Greenock to have it re-stowed. On Christmas Eve the *Irex* sailed again, but she was soon driven by another gale to take shelter in Belfast Lough, where she was forced to remain until New Year's Day, that day she left sheltered waters for the last time.

Three Weeks of Gale Force Winds

The following day found the *Irex* crashing through head on seas into another south-westerly gale with violent squalls and heavy rain. Hutton was determined to see this weather through. He had no idea that the storm would last for over three weeks and drive him out of his mind. On January 5th an enormous sea broke over the ship, six men were injured, two with broken limbs. On the 16th, the winds rose to hurricane force and remained that way for the next 10 days. Driven to the limits of exhaustion, the desperate crew asked the First Mate Irvine to seize command from Hutton, and run her into port. "I'll sink her first " he replied.

On January 23rd, the crew went straight to the Captain and requested, perhaps demanded, that he run for port. Hutton told them that he had no idea of the ship's location, thanks to the

weather, but at noon he learned his position (in the Bay of Biscay) from a passing steamer. The tired ship turned around and ran for Falmouth, which she reached at 8 p.m. the next day.

For 12 hours she rolled heavily, waiting for a pilot, but none would venture out in such a storm. When Hutton raised sail he aimed for Portland, but he had almost no idea of his true position. Mist and rain blinded the ship and added misery to the driving wind.

Captain Loses His Senses

For another 14½ hours the *Irex* aimlessly ploughed the broken windswept seas, then a light was seen on the port bow. As Hutton strained his tired eyes to see it, his mind began to play terrible tricks. He had not been to bed for 24 days and he began to hallucinate, instead of the warning red flash of the Needles Light he imagined the bright light of a pilot boat. A lookout reported land and told Hutton that they could not weather the point. "Then we must go somewhere else," the demented Captain replied, and ordered the helm straight towards the light, and the waiting rocks. Other seamen approached him and asked him to heave-to for the night, but this impertinence snapped his temper. He swore, "behaved like a madman," and ordered them to get a rope and ladder for the pilot, while he solemnly waved the binnacle lamp over his head.

A few minutes later the 400 foot cliffs of Scratchells Bay reared ahead. Hutton snapped to his senses, "Put the helm down! Brace the yards up!" but it was too late. Carried forward on the Atlantic rollers the noble steel prow smashed three times on the shallow chalk bed of the bay; and stuck rigid. The sea immediately began to flood the ruptured hull, smashed onto the stern and ran along the decks. Hutton gave orders to abandon ship immediately. The crew waded up to where he and Irvine were cutting loose one of the aft lifeboats. Irvine clambered in to find the plug, suddenly the stern was buried under a huge sea. The two aft boats were ripped from their davits and washed away. Hutton probably died instantly. Irvine was carried away yelling for help until his boat was swamped.

Shocked and terrified the crew stampeded to the nearest rigging and ascended the masts, some badly injured. The boatswain, Hanson, had the foresight to try and rescue the ship's log book from Hutton's cabin, but another sea swamped the stern, drowning Hanson and destroying the records.

Through the long foul night the desperate survivors clung to the ropes and spars with only a few blankets, some condensed milk and port wine for sustenance. Below them the deck was being swept from stern to bow. Seaman Dick Stearne had to be left on the deck all night, trapped between a winch and a spar, with a broken arm and leg. "To hear his fearful, agonising cries would have made you pity him."

The wreck was spotted at about 9 a.m. from the Needles Battery, a small fortress hewn from the chalk at the western extremity of the Island. The *Irex* lay about 300 yards offshore, her torn sails billowing in the wind. At 10 a.m. news reached Totland and soon the lifeboat *Charles Luckombe* was launched. Seeing her flares, the steam collier *Hampshire* put back and took her in tow. The rescue rocket team was summoned from Freshwater Bay and soon the downs were crowded with hundreds of anxious onlookers.

Back on board the ordeal became too much for the cabin boy, Oglivie. Ignoring the shouts of the crew he descended to the deck and sat under the hatch covers until they were all washed away. As he swam across the deck he was crushed under a spar, both his legs were broken. He finally drowned in the main hatch.

Lifeboat Rescue Fails

At 11.45 the *Hampshire* and *Charles Luckombe* arrived off the Needles, both being swept by heavy seas. At 12.23 the lifeboat let go and began to row the 300 yards to the wreck. The wrecked mariners raised a hoarse cheer and feebly waved their sodden blankets. They assumed that the lifeboat could at least save Harry Grayson, who had been left in the crew house with a broken leg. The lifeboat battled 100 yards closer in 20 minutes, but her crew became apprehensive. When a huge sea swept over her dissension broke out among the crew. Some wanted to go on "and would have risked anything" but Coxswain Stone sided with the majority, and the boat began to back away, to the dismay of the hundreds of spectators. "Are we Englishmen to leave those poor fellows clinging to the rigging?" shouted one coastguard, but the silent coxswain prevailed. Ten minutes later a huge sea smashed through the crewhouse taking Grayson with it. "He washed about on the deck for a while then got his finishing stroke through being thrown against the poop." The lifeboat watched developments, nearly being smashed under the *Hampshire's* stern, and was then towed back to her station. Dishonoured, the coxswain was replaced in a year by one of those who had urged him on.

The only hope now lay with the rocket apparatus which had arrived at the fort at 1 a.m., ten minutes later Coastguard Hallett was aiming the rocket's nose at the wreck, 300 yards out, 400 feet down and straight into the teeth of the gale. It seemed impossible but Hallett's very first shot soared down and snarled in the fore-rigging. Seaman Niccolls carried it up to the fore topmast and the rest of the crew began to work their way forward along the mainstays that connected the masts. On this perilous journey, apprentice Hatchett's numb fingers lost their grip on the cold rope and he fell to the deck below, being washed overboard. The remaining crew gathered their feeble strength and began to haul in the rope and set up the hawser, it took them two hours.

Back at the fort, this time was used to make splices and twist together every available yard of rope to cover the enormous distance. At one stage a slack rope caught under a rock at the base of the cliff, Coastguard Mayo immediately volunteered to free it.

As he descended the others tried to work it free from above. All the time the roaring gale drove shingle and pieces of chalk into the faces of the rescuers, it was almost impossible to see. Anyone who knows that cliff, and can imagine the conditions, will realise how incredibly brave Mayo was. Just as he reached the bottom the rope worked free.

When the Bosun's Chair was ready, the crew elected Niccolls to test the ropes, with the injured to follow. To the cheers of hundreds of people Niccolls was hauled to safety at 3 p.m. Next came Stearne, who had been trapped on the poop overnight — he died later in the fort. Pulling each seaman up the steep gradient, over the wild thundering waters, was exhausting work, so the gates of the fort were opened to the onlookers. Volunteers eagerly grabbed the ropes and heaved away for five hours, despite being soaked and blistered. "Pull away lads, we're lifesaving!" cheerfully shouted Chief Coastguard Spilman. His energy and confidence were infectious. Darkness fell but the work went on. The numbers pulling began to fall through exhaustion, cold and hunger, but at 8 p.m. a detachment of troops arrived from Golden Hill Fort, relieved by further reinforcements at 10.30 p.m.

Petrified Boy Lashed to the Mast

At 9.25 p.m. the 23rd man was hauled ashore. he reported six men left in the foremast, and one lad, Jones, so frightened, that he could not move from the mizzenmast. The last of the six men were hoisted ashore at 12.30, abandoning Jones, wrapped in a rug and lashed to the mast.

Through another windswept night the hull and masts held firm. In the morning, Coastguard Machin and a negro seaman, Isaac Rose, volunteered to go back for the boy. They were hoisted down to the battered, creaking wreck and descended the mast. Picking his moment, Rose sprinted to the mizzenmast, only just missing being swept away. He found Jones "blue with cold and half dead" and carried him piggy-back to the deck. In the final desperate sprint to the foremast they were buried by a charging wave, but somehow they clung on and climbed the mast to safety. Soon after

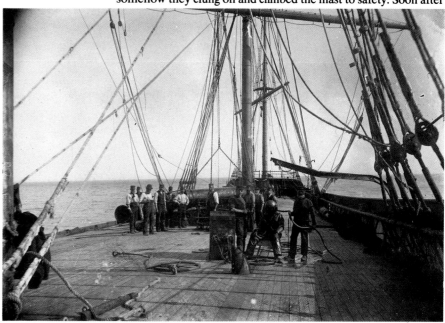

The deck of the Irex during salvage operations. (Courtesy of Eric Toogood).

the three came ashore, the line parted. They were lucky, Jones was revived and recovered, bringing the total saved to 29.

Royal Congratulations

A few days later the survivors were invited to see the Queen at Osborne House, along with the N.C.O.'s from the Needles Fort. Back in Freshwater, ugly rumours went around suggesting mutiny. The full truth will never be known, but no evidence appeared for it at the inquest on Irvine's body, or the Board of Trade Inquiry. The wreck of the *Irex* was dismantled and scrapped. Some of her timbers were used in building Irex Cottages in Clayton Road, Freshwater. The rest of her rusting hull and broken cargo still lie in the Bay.

1890-1892

Between the wrecks of the *Irex* in 1890 and the *Eider* in 1892 there were six shipwrecks including two terrible tragedies. This time also saw the setting up of a new lifeboat station, at Atherfield, in response to the *Sirenia* disaster.

On Easter Sunday, 1890, no less than four ships were embayed on the south-west coast. Luckily for the brigantine *Tyne*, Maurice Wheeler boarded the ship and guided the ship's master so that the brig escaped "literally by the skin of her teeth."

Less lucky was the schooner *Dizzy Dunlop* which went aground on the rocks at Atherfield. The Brighstone boat *Worcester Cadet* discovered that four of the crew had been rescued by the coast-guard's rocket but that the Master and Mate had stayed on. Coxswain James Cotton persuaded them to abandon her. The schooner soon broke up under the battering of the seas.

When the *Worcester Cadet* returned to station at 1 a.m., she immediately re-launched to two more wrecks on 'Shipledge.' The crew of the Penzance ketch *Cameo* made their own escape, so the lifeboat went out to the schooner *Carbocen*. Just as her Captain was welcoming the lifeboat alongside, a life saving rocket launched by the coastguards shot just past his head.

On the afternoon of October 19th, 1891, a vicious south-westerly gale embayed two French brigs. The *Henri Leontine,* was beaten ashore on Brook ledge where her six crew were rescued by a party of men led by Captain Seely. The other brig, the *Jeanne Benoni,* managed to get as far as St. Catherine's Race, despite having her jib boom torn away by the wind, but then she was struck by three enormous seas that broke clear across her deck and pushed her onto her side, sweeping away five of the six crew. Out of control, the brig swung into the wind and came ashore stern first under the lighthouse. The Blackgang rocket crew were soon on the scene, having to dismantle a wall en-route thanks to a locked gate.

The third rocket was secured by the lone survivor in the rigging. Unfortunately he did not pull out enough rope, so he found himself dangling in the air half way to safety, being thrown against the boulders around him by the furious seas. Coastguard George Haynes saved him by climbing out through the wilderness of slippery broken stone and thundering surf to cut him down. The Frenchman was saved but his ship was "smashed to atoms" and scattered for miles along the shore. The French government later awarded both Haynes and Seely medals for their "outstanding gallantry."

A few days later on October 29th, the newly formed Atherfield lifeboat crew sailed their new boat, named after its donor, *Catherine Swift,* to their recently opened station. The technical difficulties of getting the boat to the beach had been resolved by building a 240 foot rail which was tightly secured to the 75 foot cliff face. The boat descended by winch and was turned on the beach on greased timbers. To launch, the crew hauled on a rope anchored in the bay and were pushed from behind with a launching pole. Rufus and David Cotton, of *Sirenia* fame, were the two Coxswains.

At the end of that winter, in March, 1892, a Cornish brig, the *Gudrun,* went ashore on the western end of the Shingles during a severe westerly gale. She delayed showing distress signals for two hours so that it was dark by the time the Totland lifeboat, the *Charles Luckombe,* was struggling out towards her. When she finally reached the spot where the *Gudrun* had been, the brig had disintegrated. Only three of the six bodies of her crew were ever recovered.

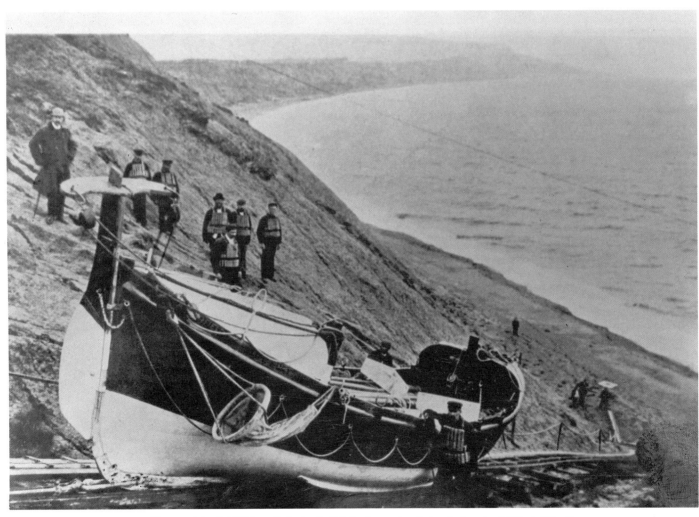

The new Atherfield lifeboat Catherine Swift being lowered to the beach along her 240 foot cliff rail.

The Eider Story

Of all the ships that came ashore on the back of the Wight there was none so spectacular, and no rescue so thoroughly successful, as that of the German luxury liner the *S.S. Eider*. She was bigger than any previous shipwreck, a four masted, two funnelled screw steamer with a gross weight of 4,719 tons and a hull over 430 feet long. Her cargo was equally unusual. Along with a crew of 167 she carried 227 passengers, 500 sacks of mail and eight and a half tons of silver and gold. For the lifeboatmen of the Western Wight she presented a challenge beyond anything in their previous experience and one to which they responded magnificently.

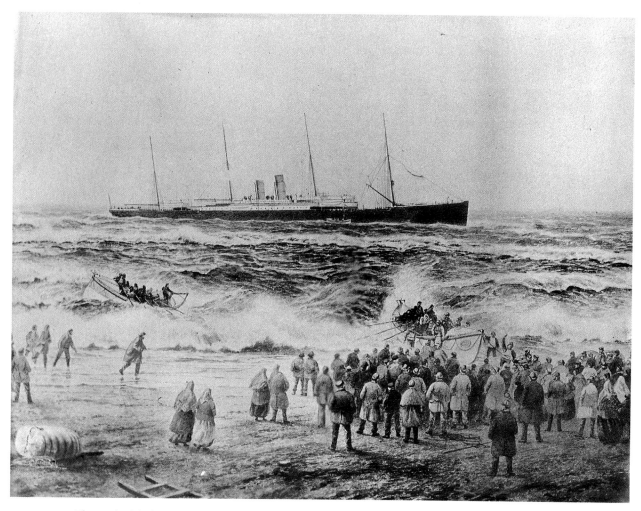

The wreck of the liner Eider, a painting by George Gregory. (Courtesy of the Longshoremen's Museum, Ventnor).

On Sunday, January 31st, 1892, the Nord-deutscher liner *S.S. Eider* was heading up the Channel through a thick fog on her regular route from New York to her home port, Bremen. She was an iron ship built at Glasgow eight years previously. She had a loading capacity of 6,000 tons or accommodation for over 1,000 passengers and yet her sleek hull could cut the waves at 16 knots.

Captain Hienecke was not too concerned about the dense fog that blinded his navigation instruments throughout the day. He was pretty sure of his course and had men taking regular soundings with the lead. As the evening drew on many of the *Eider's* officers went below to the ornate and richly decorated saloon, where the ship's orchestra was giving a grand concert for the first class passengers.

At about 10 p.m. the cut glass of the chandeliers and decanters started to rattle and clatter. There was a series of slight jerks and bumps; the officers politely excused themselves and some of the passengers went onto the promenade and boat decks. It was evident that the ship was aground but Captain Hienecke was sure that his liner would ride off with the ebbing tide. The passengers returned to their seats and the band played on.

In fact the situation was much more serious than anyone on board would have guessed. The great liner was hard aground on a worn old rock called Black Slopper, one of the many ship killing outcrops of the dreaded Atherfield Ledge.

Captain Hienecke ordered the jettisoning of some of the cargo of cotton bales and maize but the rocks refused to release their new captive. As the tide fell the 430 foot hull became more firmly embedded in the mud and rock beneath her.

Having lured the great ship onto the treacherous ledge the fog suddenly lifted, to the dumbfounded amazement of those on shore. "It looked like a town on the rocks," said one. "Well do I remember the night" wrote Fred Mew, "The firing of the guns and rockets from both ship and lifeboat station, the shouts of people running towards the cliffs, and the brilliantly lighted-up ship." Soon the crowd on the cliff were cheering the new Atherfield lifeboat, the *Catherine Swift,* as she pulled out through the rolling groundswell on her first mission of mercy.

Hienecke graciously refused Coxswain Rufus Cotton's offer of help, asking instead for tugs, but the coastguards and lifeboatmen kept a close watch on the *Eider* as the night progressed. The Atlantic swell and the wind were increasing ominously. The liner was twisting about as the water pulled her one way and another, she eventually cradled herself between two ledges of rock and lay broadside on to the sea. At 7 a.m. the *Catherine Swift* launched again and went alongside for another parley. It was already getting dangerous for anyone to try and board the lifeboat as she rose and fell by the liner's black hull. Cotton warned the ship's officers that the wind would increase into a severe gale, but Hienecke still put his faith in the tugs that were heading towards Atherfield under full steam from the Solent. The lifeboat returned ashore with some mailbags.

The Gathering Storm

As the morning progressed the gale did worsen. It was found to be impossible for the tugs to get close enough for fear of being dashed on the rocks, and by 10 a.m. Hienecke decided that the passengers must be evacuated. However, it was now too rough to launch the *Catherine Swift*. Brighstone and Brook stations were alerted and immediately proceeded to launch into the huge rollers that were now thundering along the whole line of the south-west coast and breaking against the side of the stricken steamer. Her strained iron hull groaned as she settled lower into the water.

The first lifeboat to arrive was the Brighstone boat, the *Worcester Cadet*, under Coxswain James Cotton, the brother of Tom Cotton, who had been drowned with Moses Munt during the *Sirenia* disaster. They took off a dozen women and children and beat back to the beach at Atherfield to await the lifeboat's carriage which was being brought down from Grange Chine.

The Brook boat, *William Slaney Lewis,* had a tougher struggle against adverse winds and towering seas. With the experienced hand of John Hayter at the helm and Ben Jacobs at his side, the Brook boat battled to reach the liner for five hours. The crew were continually drenched by bitterly cold February seas and many onlookers feared that she would be swamped and capsized. They watched the little boat being tossed about by the great waves "only visible when she rose on the crest of a big sea." Eventually the lifeboat reached the relatively sheltered waters of the liner's lee side and took off another load of women and children.

Women and Children First

As the Brook boat turned for shore, the *Catherine Swift*, was at last able to rush into the leaping icy surf and slowly clawed out towards the wreck meeting each incoming breaker in a violent cloud of spray. "It seemed at times that she must be driven back," but the Atherfield men held her course until they reached the calmer lee waters of the *Eider*.

By 2 p.m. it was beginning to look as if the big liner would break up as great Atlantic rollers broke over her stern. However, by 3 p.m. the wind had fallen somewhat and the three lifeboats were able to begin the evacuation in earnest. Both carriages had now arrived and had been lowered over the cliffs by the launchers and helpers. Altogether the three boats made 18 perilous trips that day. By nightfall the *William Slaney Lewis* had brought 90 people ashore, the *Worcester Cadet* 88 more and some of the mail, and the *Catherine Swift* a further 55 people and more mail.

As the passengers were helped out of the boats they were mostly drenched, frozen and exhausted. Luckily there were plenty of willing hands to lead them up the muddy paths of Shepherds Chine to the shelter of the coastguard station and the lifeboat house. The coastguards wives took many of them into their cottages and others were taken by road to Chale Rectory, Brook House and other private houses. Dry clothing was in short supply but enough food was available thanks to the generosity of the grocer of Chale who sent almost all of his provisions up the road to Atherfield. Once recovered, the passengers were sent off to Southampton where they resumed their interrupted journey to Bremen on another Nord-deutscher ship.

There was no such rest for the blistered and exhausted crews of the three lifeboats. They woke on the Tuesday morning to find that the gale had increased to storm force. The three boats had to be launched into huge breaking seas and a tearing headwind which often unleashed showers of stinging hailstones from an angry grey sky.

The *Catherine Swift* had a particularly tough launch. "Time after time she was carried back by the waves, being tossed about like a cork. In one instance her bow was lifted high up in the air and she seemed to stand erect on her stern. Then with an alarming sweep, the fore part of the boat flew over and crashed into the water, head landward and close to the beach. The spectators stood almost breathless during the struggles of the crew in the breakers, and sent up a ringing cheer when the boats head again put to sea." Even when the lifeboat reached the *Eider*, Rufus did not allow anyone to board her for almost half an hour, as he considered the risks of being swamped or capsized were far too great. By now the wreck

was badly holed and sinking deeper under the weight of water in her hold, the stern promenade submerged beneath the incensed white waves.

Despite the appalling conditions the rescue work went on until all 146 of the remaining crew and all the remaining mail bags had been brought ashore in 11 perilous trips, all without a single casualty.

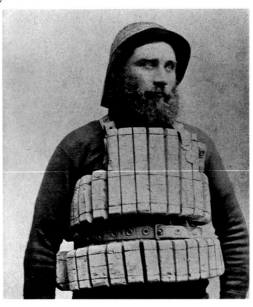

James Cotton, Coxswain of the Brighstone lifeboat for 27 years from 1887. He received the R.N.L.I. Silver Medal for his part in the Eider rescue. (Courtesy of Geoffrey Cotton).

With all 379 people safely ashore by Tuesday night, attention now switched to the £300,000 worth of gold and silver sitting in the *Eider's* vault. With the consent of the R.N.L.I. the lifeboatmen accepted the offer of reward money and over the next two days the tough longshoremen ran up a final total of 41 trips to the *Eider* as they brought ashore all the silver and gold, the ship's silver plate, and all the passenger's luggage, earning £543 in all. The precious metal was handed over to heavily armed coastguards on the beach.

Royal Thanks and Bullion Reward

On the Wednesday night the secretaries of the three lifeboat stations received a message of warm appreciation from Queen Victoria and on Friday the Prince of Wales and Prince George personally congratulated Rufus Cotton and Charles Dabell, secretary of the local lifeboat committee.

This remarkable rescue was hailed by the press not only in Britain but around the world. Tributes and congratulations were offered by individuals and institutions from many countries. The German Emperor, Wilhelm II, presented each of the coxswains with a gold watch inscribed with his personal commendation for their outstanding courage. The R.N.L.I. honoured many of those involved, James Cotton received a Silver Medal, while Rufus Cotton and John Hayter received a second and third service clasp to their Silver Medals.

It was probably the most glorious time in the history of the Back of the Wight, and an auspicious opening in the career of the Atherfield station. It was also the moment that John Hayter chose to retire after serving for 32 years as the Brook Coxswain, during which time the crews under his command had saved 222 lives. Hayter was the most highly decorated lifeboatman in the Island's history. He was succeeded by his Second Coxswain, Ben Jacobs.

As the main British salvage companies refused Nord-deutschers offers of a contract, thanks to the reputation of Atherfield Ledge, it went to a small Scandinavian company, Neptun Salvage. They slaved over the wreck for two months, working night and day to pump her out and patch her wounds. According to the company's records it took "a giant effort" using portable steam pumps and four vessels to get the great ship to move from her bed of mud and rock. The *Eider* was finally hauled off the ledge on March 29th and towed to Southampton. However, she was in such a state that Nord-deutscher declared that she was a total loss and on December 13th, 1892, she went under the hammer at an auction at Lloyds in London.

The Alcester

Following the wrecks of the *Irex* and the *Eider* the only other big wreck of the nineties was the Liverpool registered, full rigged *Alcester,* which was lost on Atherfield Ledge in February, 1897.

The *Alcester* was completed at Greenock in 1883 and was owned by a Mrs. Haws, and commanded by her son, Captain Allison Haws. She was iron built and weighed 1,596 tons. Her hull was 257 feet long and she carried a crew of 24.

October, 1896, found the *Alcester* in the bustling port of Calcutta where she was loaded with 2,360 tons of jute, a plant fibre used to make cordage and baggage. On November 2nd she raised sail in the Bay of Bengal and began the long journey to Hamburg. After an uneventful voyage she reached the Channel in the early hours of February 19th. Captain Haws took a bearing from Start Point but then lost sight of the land as his ship was surrounded by a thickening mist. At 3.30 p.m. the *Alcester* was swallowed up by a particularly dense fog bank. At 4 p.m. Haws checked his depth and went below to the Chart Room. Having carefully estimated his position as past St. Catherine's he ordered the helm north-east by east but on returning to the deck he was shocked to see that the water was yellow, meaning land close by. The wheel was spun hard to port but to no avail, and with all the momentum of her 6,000 tons riding the sea at six to seven knots, the *Alcester's* majestic bow ploughed onto Typit Ledge. Fog and tide had lured yet another victim onto the rocks at Atherfield.

The *Catherine Swift* was launched at 7 p.m. and soon reached the big ship out in the fog. Haws declined the offer of help but asked Coxswain Rufus Cotton to send a telegram for tugs. He should have asked the lifeboatmen to take out anchors to secure his stern or used one of his own boats, as when the sun rose over a clear sea the following morning, the ocean swell had driven the *Alcester* broadside onto the shore, closer in, and hard aground. When the Lloyds agent went aboard with some longshoremen Haws told them that the hull was badly strained and making water but that he expected to be towed off later that day. At about 9 a.m. a tug arrived and after making a salvage deal with Haws her Master fixed up a hawser and began to drag the great full rigger back towards safe waters.

The *Alcester's* hull groaned and screeched as she was pulled across her unyielding mattress of rock. The strained hawser snapped and the partially floated ship was carried further in by the swell. Throughout the morning the tug's big engines fought to save the protesting hull from the hungry grip of the rocks but two more hawsers parted and the ship was driven onto the ledge more firmly than ever. Her hull settled on a big gnarled rock under her midships. This ripped a hole in her iron skin so that she rapidly filled with water and settled deeper into the growing Atlantic swell. At noon the tug gave up on its hopeless task and steamed away from the storm that her skipper could feel was on its way. The ship's crew were also getting worried by the growing size of the incoming rollers and asked Haws to signal for the lifeboat, which he did at 1 p.m.

The Stubborn Captain

The rescue of the crew took most of the afternoon. The *Catherine Swift* made two trips and brought ashore 22 men and their belongings; a cat, a dog and two monkeys. Rufus Cotton and the Lloyds agent did their best to convince Haws to leave the ship but he was determined to remain with her, despite the fact that the wet cargo of Jute was swelling in the holds, forcing up the decks and bursting the beams with a sound like a pistol shot. His faithful First Mate decided to stay too. The stubborn Captain rejected their warnings of an imminent storm. This was his mother's only ship and he was determined to stay with it. The two men went below to work out the crew's wages but after a time the sea was making such a disturbing sound that they went on deck and found themselves trapped in a howling storm. "It was frightful up there . . . the sea all around was like a snowfield."

As the seas began to crash onto the poop the two men retreated to the foc'sle and then up to the fore-top, the platform halfway up the foremast. They loosed the topgallant sail and cut it to make a shelter from the gale. At 9 p.m. Haws burned a blue light as a signal

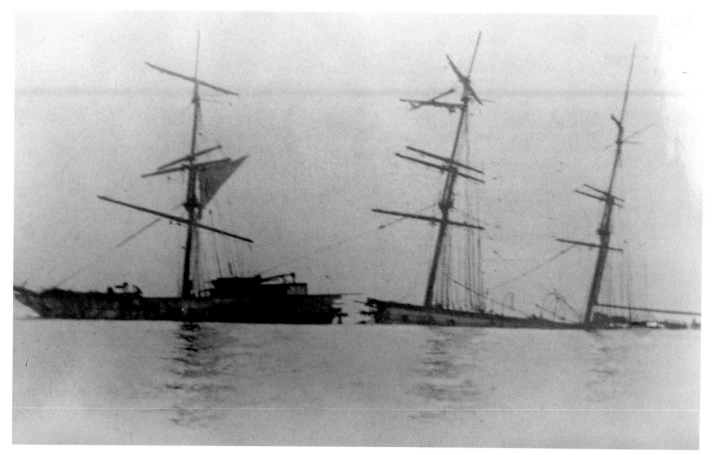

The full rigged Alcester photographed after the final rescue of the Captain and Mate.

to the lifeboat but the valiant attempt to launch was a failure. "By this time it was high water and quite impossible for the boat to be launched, as the seas were sweeping the foot of the slipway and there was not room to turn the boat on the shore."

Night's Ordeal: Trapped in the Fore-Top

The two men aboard the *Alcester* realised that they would have to wait until the morning and as the waves and the wind rose higher their prospects of living that long diminished rapidly. Haws later recalled the night's ordeal in a letter to his mother. "The seas were coming over aft and sweeping right forward over the bows smashing and destroying all in their way. One sea came over and washed away lifeboats aft and bridge, all in one smash." This left only one lifeboat. The Mate wanted to take it but Haws told him that they would not even reach the surf alive, "it would look well in the morning to find us both drowned and the masts standing alright."

By eleven o'clock Haws and the Mate were facing certain death. "It was blowing very hard and everything seemed to be breaking up. We both thought we were done for so I said to the Mate: "I hope you will forgive me for causing you to lose your life by remaining with the ship." "Don't let that lay on your mind sir" replied his fatalistic companion, "I have no-one to look to me, you have a wife and children." The Mate then curled up under the mast to sleep and "forget my misery." Haws covered him with the torn sail and sat puffing his way through a dozen fat cigars while he worked out an escape plan which involved sliding down the thick ropes that run to the bowsprit, in case the foremast should fall.

Thankfully the conditions began to improve after midnight as the tide fell and the gale lost some of its blind fury. By the morning the decks were safe to walk and the two haggard men descended from their wooden perch. They found the ship in a complete shambles. "Such a scene of desolation I never saw. I have seen a few ships that have been cleaned by hurricanes in the East Indies, but this beat all. We could not help laughing at the way the inside of the forecastle was cleaned out." Even the stove had been swept from the cookhouse.

"Jump For Your Lives!"

Back on shore Rufus and his men had waited up all night for a sufficient break in the weather and now they began pushing the *Catherine Swift* towards the thundering surf on its greased timbers. The wind was still blowing strong from the south-west with great rollers still running across the bay, but the launch was a success. The lifeboat then rowed and sailed far out to sea before turning to pick up a lift from the incoming swell. As the lifeboat approached the forlorn wreck Cotton yelled out "Jump! Jump for your lives!" They needed no persuading. They leapt from the ship into the lifeboat "full of thanks for the crew that had dared so much for them."

"We got ashore alright amidst much cheering from the people lining the cliffs. As the Mate said we were stared at like wild animals. No doubt we looked a sight."

The whole crew had been saved but the ship and its cargo were completely lost. A couple of hours after the final rescue the ship broke in two. By the afternoon the top of the mainmast had gone and a lot of the ship and its cargo was washing up in the surf. The Lloyds agent went aboard her the following day but left immediately as the forced up decks made him feel sick.

Captain Haws was tried by a Board of Trade Inquiry held at Greenock in March. It was found that he did not use his lead enough and he had his Master's Licence suspended for three months. He had also lost his possessions with the ship but at least he was alive and that he owed to the lifeboat crew of Atherfield.

As usual the local people tried to salvage the ships miserable remains from the sea, and the coastguards tried to stop them, at least most did. One day young Fred Mew and a friend were climbing Ladder Chine with bundles of wood when they saw a coastguard approaching. They dropped the bundles and chatted to the officer. "He then strolled to the edge of the cliff and looking over he saw 15 people coming up with loads. He at once turned to us with a wink and said 'I must be going, Ladder is no place for me!' . . as he stepped over the bank he stumbled over one of our two loads . . . he burst out laughing, and said 'Goodnight.' By the way, he was a native of the Island; and that speaks for itself.

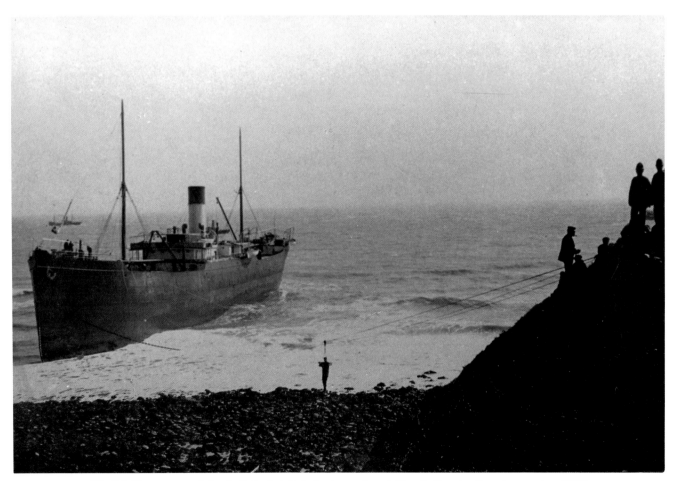

The S.S. Moyunne stranded at St. Catherine's Point but later refloated. Note the Breeches Buoy in operation. (1897).

The Turn of the Century: 1898-1902

The close of the Victorian era saw the Island's sea rescue services at their peak, with five R.N.L.I. stations and a coastguard now given over almost completely to shipping observation and inshore rescue. This time also saw the end of the period of frequent shipwrecks and rescues as steam further replaced sail and tugs saved the bulk of the casualties without incident. However, there remained some notable exceptions.

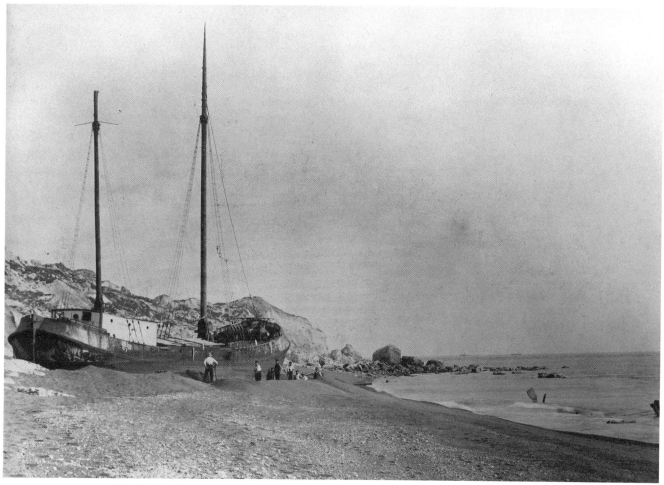

The Dutch galliot Mathilde, high and dry on the beach beneath Blackgang Chine, November, 1898.

In November, 1898, the weather was particularly vicious, lashing the base of the Island's crumbling cliffs, destroying two ships, and nearly beaching a steamer. Fred Mew recalled November 23rd clearly. "For many hours the wind blew a gale from the south accompanied by driving rain and there was a particularly heavy sea running in Chale Bay." After lunch, Fred's father called him outside to see three ships being driven towards the shore. Both men dressed up and rushed towards the cliff. The force of the wind was terrific. "At times it was a case of holding onto the gorse bushes to prevent oneself from being blown down."

One of the sailing ships just managed to get around the point at St. Catherine's but the smaller one, the Dutch galliot *Mathilde* was washed high onto the beach under Blackgang. The other vessel, the steamer *Huntcliffe,* disabled by the storm, saved herself by dropping her anchors just a few hundred yards from the shore. She was able to crawl away the following day, just missing the Atherfield Ledge on her outward journey.

Salvage Struggle for the Mathilde

The *Mathilde's* crew were brought to safety by the Wheeler family. Local men were later employed to carry her cargo of white oats to the top of the cliff and in the sad job of dismantling the ship. The man who bought her hulk had an unfortunate time. While he was preparing her salvage, a huge sea removed her to St. Catherine's where the whole process of salvage began again. The hulk was lifted by hydraulic jacks onto massive baulks of timber from which it could be launched into the sea. However, the ocean returned to claim her prize, removed the whole assembly, and smashed the galliot hulk to pieces along the southern cliffs. Weeks of work and a lot of money disappeared that night.

German Schooner Smashed on Shingles

The other victim of this terrible November weather was the German three masted schooner *Ernst.* Captain Willis and his crew fought valiantly to get the *Ernst* into the shelter of the Solent during a violent storm that built up to hurricane force, with winds of over 70 miles an hour lashing the sea into a frenzy. Huge racing seas charged from the obscured southern horizon, their crested tops torn away by the wind and thrown through the air. The doomed ship was beaten onto the western end of the Shingles, where she was seen by the coastguards who alerted the lifeboat station at Totland.

The Totland crew had never been out in conditions like this, and darkness had long since fallen when the *Charles Luckombe* swept down her ramp at 9.20 p.m. It took a long time to reach the wrecks' location and then find her. The lifeboatmen were almost blinded by flying spray which struck their faces like a whiplash. Visibility was appalling. When they found the *Ernst* it was impossible to go alongside. The seas were so heavy that the lifeboat would have been grounded in the hollow of a wave, or thrown onto the Shingles where the crew would have been killed in seconds. The great shoal was causing the waves to explode upwards, pillars of water being thrown into the air by the extraordinary pressure of ocean being crushed against rock. For about an hour the *Charles Luckombe* pitched and rolled in this nightmare world, unable to do anything for the wretched crew of the *Ernst,* who were clinging onto dear life as their ship buckled and cracked under the heaving weight of the sea.

At midnight Coxswain Simmonds shouted to his men to row back to Totland to telegraph for a tug. This done, the oarsmen pulled the lifeboat back to the scene of the wreck, and anchored to leeward to await events.

At 6 a.m. the hull of the schooner finally collapsed and she quickly splintered to pieces. The lifeboat pulled towards the sound of the cries of the drowning crew. Captain Willis was rescued from a piece of wreckage, and the Mate and a seaman were pulled from a water-filled boat. They were exhausted and close to death. For a further hour the lifeboat searched the area, but no trace of the other six men or the ship could be found.

When the boat was winched back into her boathouse Simmonds received a new message. Four of the *Ernst's* crew had been seen drifting on a flat piece of wreckage towards Christchurch. The lifeboat launched again. The hurricane winds had passed, but there was still a heavy groundswell left in their wake. The tired Totland crew searched for over five hours they found nothing. When they returned to station it was noted that but they had been out for 16 hours in some of the worst weather that Island lifeboatmen had ever had to face. If they were disheartened by their failure to find the four men, their humour was restored by the news that they had reached Christchurch after an unusual voyage on the cookhouse roof.

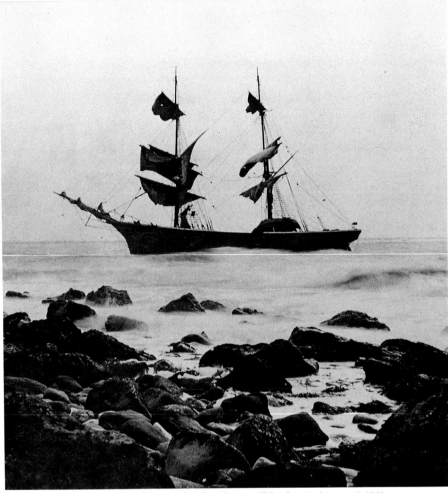

The wreck of the smuggling brig Russie off Rocken End in April, 1902.

Bembridge Rescues

The Bembridge lifeboat *Queen Victoria* went to the aid of two shipwrecks in 1899.

In January the Calais schooner *Rosalie* grounded on Bembridge Ledge in a strong west-north-westerly gale. By the time the *Queen Victoria* reached her she was badly holed and full of water. The crew of five men and a boy were brought ashore at 11.30 p.m.

In December the *Queen Victoria* rescued a future admiral of the Grand Fleet, then Commander Beatty, whose naval torpedo boat *059* had grounded on the ledge. The 14 crew were brought ashore while their vessel was left to the naval salvage tugs.

Beatty later led the battlecruiser squadron at the Battle of Jutland in 1916, the biggest naval battle in history, and he received the surrender of the German fleet in 1918.

Near Disaster on Atherfield Ledge

One of the most dramatic rescues in the history of the Back of the Wight took place on February 15th, 1900. The German barque *Auguste,* a three masted iron ship bound from Australia to London with a cargo of Jarrah wood was caught in a tremendous southerly gale.

Captain Ammerman and his 18 crew were off course and had little idea of where they were. Visibility had been reduced to a minimum by violent squalls and driving rain. When Ammerman briefly saw the shore near Ladder Chine he tried to put the ship about, but the 1,300 ton barque was not that nimble. Instead she grounded stern first on the eastern side of the Atherfield Ledge, with her bows facing into the growing tempest.

The ship grounded at 4.30 p.m. but it was another hour before the *Catherine Swift* was able to launch into that terrible sea. By then the crew of the barque were up in the rigging as the decks were being swept by the waves.

Valiantly Coxswain Rufus Cotton and the Atherfield crew fought to climb the big incoming seas that were being driven ever faster by the increasing gale. Whenever they made a little progress the bows of the lifeboat would be beaten back by a succession of charging breakers, pushing her off course and back towards the beach. Frequently the *Catherine Swift* was buried by the sea "it being just a miracle that they were not all washed out of her." After

repeated attempts to make headway against the onshore gale the exhausted crew returned the lifeboat to the beach.

Once ashore the lifeboatmen climbed the cliff to join the big crowd that had now gathered to watch the barque. The *Auguste* was in a bad way, with each sea breaking right over her, her tough iron hull ruptured and torn on the rocks below. It was decided to call out the Brighstone boat *Joe Jarman,* but the Brighstone crew had even less success than their comrades. The carriage twice sank into the mud, and when the boat was finally launched, some hours later, it went aground on a sandbank.

Back at Atherfield the coastguards tried firing several rescue rockets at the barque's tattered rigging but each one was picked up by the gale and cast into the sea. The people onshore were running out of ideas. A telegram was sent to Southsea requesting a tug and a lifeboat, but all could see that the wreck was unlikely to hold together until their arrival.

In the early hours of the morning the anxious onlookers felt the gale shift slightly, so it was no longer coming directly onshore. Rufus and his men seized their chance. The *Catherine Swift* was heaved off her launch ramp into the oncoming breakers at 2.30 a.m. and began to sweep out strongly to the sodden exhausted men in the *Auguste's* rigging. The waters of the eastern ledge were still a frenzy of white broken waves and flying spume, but this time the lifeboatmen had the situation in hand. The *Catherine Swift* got alongside the battered ship and took off all 18 men without injury. The crowded lifeboat returned to the beach directly opposite the wreck, to the massed cheers of the hundreds of people gathered on the cliff and shore. When Captain Ammerman and his men clambered from the boat they too began cheering. It had been a brilliant rescue. It was also the last with Rufus Cotton at the helm. In 1904 he was succeeded by Walter White, another of the heroic volunteer crew of the final *Sirenia* rescue.

The crew of the *Auguste* were taken care of in the usual way by the Shipwrecked Mariners Society, and they were able to save much of their gear and some of the cargo from their ship over the following days. The *Auguste* herself was beyond redemption, becoming yet another addition to the Atherfield ship's graveyard.

46

The Smuggling Russie

The wreck of the smuggling brig *Russie* could not provide a greater contrast to the high drama of the *Auguste* rescue. When she rammed into Rocken End on Easter Sunday, 1902, the sea was calm and twinkled in the bright sunshine. The brig was just passing St. Catherine's on the outward journey to the Newfoundland fishing grounds. The winds were light and spasmodic and the *Russie's* 31 crew had the ship under full sail. "Evidently she got a little too close to the shore in a flukey wind, which dropping suddenly, she drifted onto the rocks with all sail set."

The fine ship was doomed. Being empty she could not be lightened of her cargo. The crew almost immediately abandoned her, coming ashore in the ship's small fishing boats. The next day they brought their baggage ashore and this was searched by the coastguards. It was then that the first doubts arose over whether the *Russie* was just going on a fishing trip, as all the crew were carrying large amounts of tobacco. This was emptied into a basket. Fred Mew happened to be present and recorded that when the senior officer was called outside to discuss the fate of the ship's two dogs, the basket was quickly lightened of much of its load, the Frenchmen stuffing their pockets while the junior coastguards packed their jerseys, although they were later subtly persuaded to return it by their senior officer.

Over the next few days local longshoremen began stripping down the brig and bringing ashore the fishing gear and salt stowed in her holds. However this was not the only thing she was carrying. After a week the wind picked up and the brig was beaten against the unyielding boulders of Rocken End by the Atlantic swell, and began to break up. Then the real nature of her aborted trip became apparent as the seas were crowded with bobbing barrels of wine and spirits. Ever alert to the possible gains of a ship coming apart, the local people were soon busy tapping the barrels and climbing the cliffs with "buckets, pails and jars of every description and size." The ship's food stores also provided a ready harvest. Fish, pork, lard, butter and sausages came ashore in large quantities. However, the main source of interest, for the men at least, was the profusion of alcohol. News quickly spread and soon the remote shore was milling with a reeling crowd of pie-eyed locals. "People just fell and lay about anywhere in a state of oblivion." To stop this alcoholic orgy the coastguards came down to the shore and poured away or seized the rest of the offending spirits.

The *Russie* was soon smashed to pieces and her ramains sold. Thanks to the duty placed on the tobacco and drink confiscated by the coastguard, it could not be sold, as the local price was still subsidised by smuggling (or free trade as the Islanders preferred to call it). As a result the coastguards poured away all the drink in their custody. "What a waste" lamented Fred Mew in later years, "truly some of our laws are beyond understanding."

The Final Exploits of the Rowing Lifeboats 1904-1924

By the 1900's major shipwrecks were becoming rare and the five lifeboats sometimes stood idle for years. One station which continued to see plenty of action was Totland. Of the others, the Atherfield boat *Catherine Swift*, was crippled in 1906 and the Ryde boat, *Selina*, capsized with the loss of two lives in 1907. By 1924 the rowing lifeboats had almost disappeared thanks to the far greater range and speed of the two new motor lifeboats stationed at Bembridge and Yarmouth.

The Career of the Robert Fleming

In 1903 the station at Totland was equipped with a new lifeboat, the *Robert Fleming*. Her first call came on May 2nd, 1904, when the Cornish schooner *Saint* ran aground on Warden Ledge while seeking shelter from a violent south-westerly storm. The *Robert Fleming* slid down her long ramp at 6.30 a.m. into a heavy sea and blinding snow storm. The Totland crew took off the Captain's wife and four crew but Captain Clapet and his mate decided to stay with the ship until they were forced to make further distress signals. The Totland boat launched again to rescue them but was considerably damaged on the rocks. The *Saint* became a total wreck.

On January 22nd, 1907, the Totland boat was called out to the aid of the crew of the Southampton ketch *Effort*. She had been deliberately grounded on the Shingles so that her crew could collect a cargo of loose stone for the building industry. However, when the tide rose to refloat the ketch it was accompanied by a bitterly cold north-east gale which dashed huge waves over the ship. The five crew were seen running around on the dry part of the shoal in a desperate attempt to keep from freezing. The *Robert Fleming* launched at 5.30 p.m. but could not get too close for fear of going aground, so Coxswain Simmonds anchored the boat and veered down as close as he could. "A line was thrown to the men and by this means they were hauled into the lifeboat. It was intensely cold and the rescued men suffered greatly from the exposure, a boy being almost in a state of collapse when landed." The Hampshire men recovered the ketch the following day.

Later that year the *Robert Fleming* spent an afternoon searching for the crew of the *Rhoda*, which sank between the Needles and Swanage in a severe north-west gale. The crew of seven were never found.

Altogether the *Robert Fleming* made 30 launches during 17 years of service, saving 19 lives and assisting many ships. Coxswain Simmonds retired in 1913 after 22 years of exemplary service. In 1924 the station was moved to Yarmouth and equipped with the new motor lifeboat *BASP*.

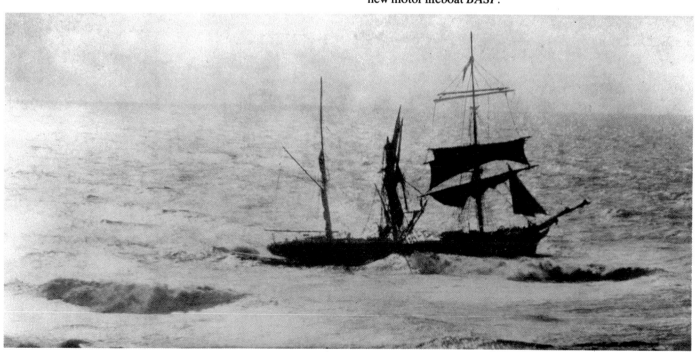

The wreck of the German barque Auguste, ashore on Atherfield Ledge in February, 1900.

The Loss of the Firefly

The last call for the *Catherine Swift* came on January 9th, 1906, in a vain effort to save the three crew of the ketch rigged *Firefly*, which lead to the crippling of the Atherfield boat.

The *Firefly* was an 82 foot iron barge "in good, seaworthy condition" which was engaged in carrying 150 tons of loose stone, bound for Langstone Harbour. She set sail from Cherbourg at midnight on January 8th in company with four other barges, similarly laden. By the following day the moderate south-westerly breeze had increased into a full gale accompanied by heavy seas and frequent squalls. By midday the little stone convoy was well scattered. In St. Catherine's Lighthouse Chief Officer Goddard could see two barges passing beneath him and the *Firefly* about three miles astern, under a reefed mainsail, foresail, jib and topsail.

The waters of St. Catherine's Race were running high that day and as she entered the steep fast running waves the ketch's bow began to rear up and crash down into the troughs, her decks awash and her sails flapping in the rain. Through his telescope Goddard could clearly see the three crew struggling to shorten sail when a huge wave errupted behind the ship and struck her on the starboard quarter, pitching the barge onto her port side. The cargo immediately shifted and the ship disappeared into the sea in a few seconds.

Goddard immediately telephoned Atherfield and the lifeboat crew were quickly summoned. They had a brief consultation with Coxswain Walter White as to whether they could launch because the lifeboat's rudder had been smashed during her quarterly exercises. They decided to go ahead, steering with the large sweep oar, and soon the lifeboat was fighting her way through the bay against a powerful headwind while being lashed by rain and pitched by the heavy swell.

As they pulled past Blackgang the lifeboatmen accepted the offer of a tow from the Southampton tug *Ajax*. She passed a warp to the lifeboat's bowman Walter Woodford, but as soon as it pulled taught it was snapped by the heavy sea. The *Ajax* went astern and passed another line to Woodford but as he was securing it a huge sea struck the *Ajax*, lifting her up and driving her stern over the lifeboat. With a great crash the tug came down on the boat, missing Woodford's head by inches, but crushing her thick bow. With the bow beaten down Woodford had to connect the line to the side of the lifeboat, so that it pulled sideways on, "every sea coming in one side and out the other, and it was only by hanging on to the lifelines and the thwarts that the crew kept in her." The lifeboat complained bitterly, creaking and cracking under the enormous strain, and Coxswain White decided to release the tow and "trust to the oars."

By the time the *Catherine Swift* reached the scene of the *Firefly's* disappearance it was 3.30 p.m. and they could find no trace of the ketch or her crew, who were probably dragged down with the ship into the chasm of St. Catherine's Deep.

As wind and tide were now driving the crippled lifeboat to the east, Coxswain White realised that his exhausted oarsmen could never make it back to Atherfield so he steered for Ventnor, and when landing there proved impossible, the boat went on to Shanklin, where she was beached with the help of local people. The crew were sent home by train and cart. As Fred Mew and his father were walking home up Southdown Road the older man said: "I never thought to see this road again boy, when we were under that tugs stern." It had been a lucky escape. After a record career, saving 158 lives in 15 years, the *Catherine Swift* was condemned. She was replaced, but the lack of wrecks in the coming years, and the constant erosion of the cliff led naturally to the closure of the station in 1915. Brighstone Grange also closed in the same year, after 55 years service, during which time her boats had saved 433 people.

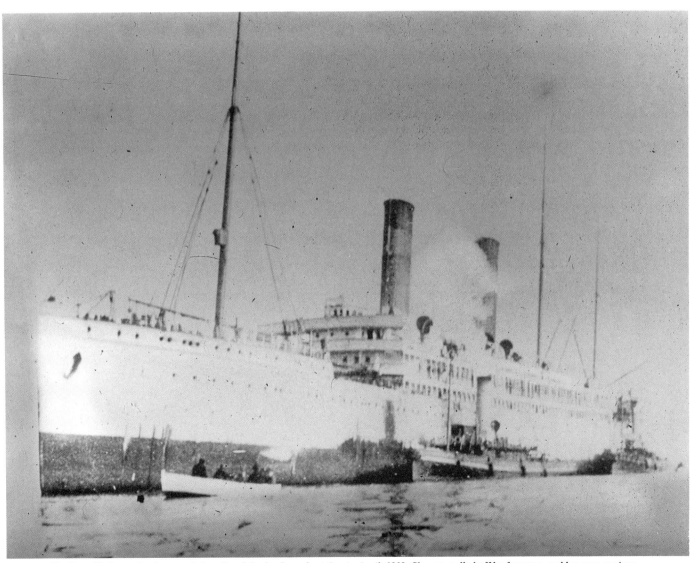

The liner Kinfauns Castle, stranded on Brook Ledge for a short time in April, 1902. She was pulled off by four tugs and her own engines.

The Selina Tragedy

A year after the crippling of the *Catherine Swift* the R.N.L.I. on the Island suffered a far greater disaster, the loss of the Ryde lifeboat *Selina,* on January 1st, 1907.

In 1905 Ryde Lifeboat Station was equipped with a new 30 foot whaleboat, the *Selina,* which was housed half way up the western side of the pier. On New Year's Day, 1907, the crew were summoned to the aid of Mr. Jarret, a barge skipper who had set off to his vessel that afternoon in a rowing dinghy. He had broken his rowlocks and was now drifting helplessly across a gale-swept Spithead.

The nine man crew of the *Selina,* under Coxswain Bartlett, launched the boat at about 5.15 p.m. It was a foul evening. The grey sea was getting rough as it was buffeted by the south-westerly gale which rose to force 9, and whipped up further by a series of violent squalls. It was already dark and visibility was further reduced by thick rain.

The lifeboat made a long search of the Spithead, firing off several flares, but there was no sign of Jarret; he washed up at Southsea at 8.30 p.m., little the worse for his ordeal. Giving up the search the *Selina* began to tack back to Ryde under reefed sails. As it approached the pier the boat was suddenly struck by a powerful gust of wind which pushed over the mast and raised a sea that capsized the boat. The crew only had time to let go the sails and jump into the icy water. The *Selina* was not a self-righting boat, so her crew had to just hang on to her bottom as she drifted before the gale.

As the hours slowly passed the nine frozen drenched men all wondered how much longer they could endure the torture of hanging on, and refuse the temptation to just let go. After two hours of this ordeal Frank Haynes gave up his benumbed grip and sank beneath the blackened surface of the Solent. Half an hour later he was followed by the Second Coxswain Henry Heward.

The seven men left were uplifted by the sight of land. An hour and a half later, the *Selina* was blown ashore at Southsea where the seven survivors were rescued by the police and coastguards. The *Selina* was not badly damaged and was soon back on station and brought up to strength by new volunteers. The R.N.L.I. gave £200 to the local fund for the families of the two drowned men which eventually reached £887.

In 1923 the Ryde station was closed as its area could be covered by the new motor lifeboat at Bembridge.

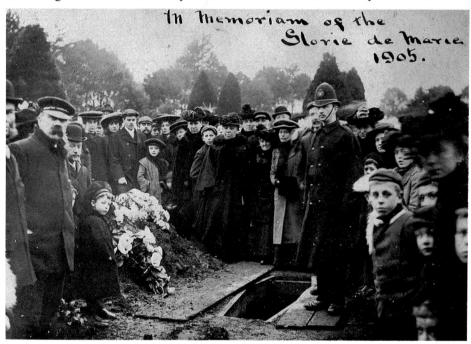

The funeral of the three crew of the French ketch Gloire de Marie. On the foul stormy morning of January 16th, 1905, they struggled around Rocken End and through St. Catherine's Race only to be driven ashore between Dunnose and Luccombe where all three quickly perished. The ketch was smashed to splinters.

The Gladiator

In April, 1908, the Royal Navy suffered two disasters off the Island's coasts when two cruisers were sunk in two separate collisions. The first was *H.M.S. Tiger* which was rammed while on manoeuvers south of St. Catherine's. The second was *H.M.S. Gladiator* which was rammed and sunk just off Yarmouth.

A mere three weeks after the loss of the *Tiger, H.M.S. Gladiator,* one of the ships that had gone to the assistance of the *Tiger* before she sank, sailed from Portland at 10.30 a.m. on April 25th, 1908, to steam up the coast to Portsmouth. The *Gladiator* was a twelve year old twin screw cruiser weighing 5,750 tons with a complement of 250 men. It was a foul day and an uncomfortable voyage, cold and misty with frequent falls of snow and a strong north-west wind.

Two hours after the *Gladiator* left Portland the American express mail liner *St. Paul* weighed anchor in Southampton Water and set off for the western Solent on her voyage to Cherbourg and then New York. She was a big ship, 11,630 tons gross, and she had 20,000 h.p. turning her screws at a rate that could push her at 21 knots. As the *St. Paul* approached Yarmouth Captain Passow reduced to half speed as visibility fell off rapidly thanks to an intense blizzard. At that moment the *Gladiator,* under Captain Lumsden was entering Hurst Race. One of the crew records the squall which struck the ship. "The snow came down thicker than ever and the wind was blowing with almost hurricane force from the north-west." Both ships were quickly blanketed in thick driven snow.

Collision off Yarmouth

The two ships did not see one another until they were less than half a mile apart, heading on a direct collision course. The *Gladiator* was moving at nine knots, the *St. Paul* at 13 knots. The men on both bridges had only seconds to react. There is a general rule that two ships meeting head-on should swing the helm hard to port, which makes the bows swing to starboard, so the two ships pass beside each other on the port side. On this occasion something went wrong. Captain Passow aboard the *St. Paul* correctly ordered the engines to stop, the helm hard to port and then the starboard engine hard astern to swing the ship. Lieutenant Mainguy, the *Gladiator's* Navigation officer ordered the helm "Port 10" but as both ships' sirens blasted almost simultaneously the officers on the bridge thought the *St. Paul* had blasted twice, which means "going to port" and the big American ship did seem to be veering that way for a moment. "Amidships. Starboard thirty" ordered Mainguy and thus both ships went on opposite tacks, the *St. Paul's* great bow heading straight for the cruiser's side. "Hard a port" shouted Lumsden but it was too late.

49

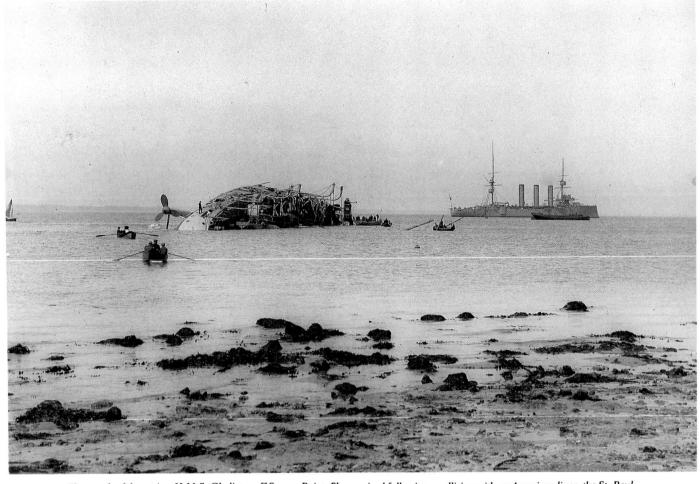

The wreck of the cruiser H.M.S. Gladiator off Sconce Point. She capsized following a collision with an American liner, the St. Paul, during an intense April blizzard. 28 of her crew perished. (Courtesy of Beken of Cowes).

At 2.29 the liner's bow crashed into the cruiser's midships with a terrible "thunderous grating noise" smashing straight into a mess room, killing several men and pinning others down. The rest of the crew were "suddenly thrown clean across the ship" and many were injured. Some of the stokers were buried in coal for a while and all the lights in the ship went out.

For a moment the two ships stood together in the blizzard while the naval ratings rescued the injured and brought them up to the deck. Then Lumsden hailed the *St. Paul* to back off. As she did so the icy sea began to rush into the huge gap torn by the liner's bow. Lumsden ordered the watertight doors to be closed and the boats to be lowered, but without success. Water still poured into the doomed warship, the starboard boats were mostly smashed by the collision and the port boats could not be lowered due to the angle of the ship as she capsized.

Luckily the gale drove the cruiser downwind and after a few minutes she grounded on Sconce Point, just west of Yarmouth, but as she drifted she rolled onto her torn starboard side throwing many of the sailors into the sea, still wearing their heavy seaboots and oilskins. Others, thinking the ship was going down, just leapt into the big breaking waves in an attempt to swim to the Island just 250 yards from where the ship finally grounded. Soon 40 or 50 men were splashing around in the freezing sea, the rest crowded along the slippery upturned side of the ship. Of the four boats that the crew managed to launch, the whaler sank immediately and the cutter made only one trip ashore before it filled with water because of the damage it suffered in the terrific sea that was then running. Those in the water were soon in trouble. The tidal current off Sconce Point is one of the most dangerous off Britain's coasts. For the moment the *St. Paul* could do nothing as Passow tried to manoeuvre her huge bulk so that her five port lifeboats could be launched in the lee of the blizzard. The crew found that the ropes and pulleys were frozen and choked with ice. It took about 20 minutes to get their boats into the water, and even then one of them was driven off by the wind.

Despite the utter desperation of the situation there was no sense of panic among the sailors, their discipline was "simply magnificent."

A great number of the *Gladiator's* crew would have drowned were it not for the prompt action and gallantry of the Royal Engineer garrison at Fort Victoria, where the cruiser had the good fortune to come aground. As soon as the soldiers realised what was happening they ran out of the fort to dash along the shore to the small pier while some broke open the boat house and launched the fort's racing gig and three dinghies. The rest simply waded in to the aid of the sailors swimming ashore, or pulled off their clothes to leap in to drag to shore those who were evidently in difficulties. "They fearlessly faced the dashing seas and at the risk of their own lives went to the succour of their comrades," reported the County Press. One, Corporal Stenning, saved seven men before he himself was carried from the sea suffering from exposure and exhaustion; and Corporal Poole swam out 150 yards to save torpedo gunner Chapman, who was drifting off in the current.

Once the poorly handled boats of the *St. Paul* arrived the evacuation of the rest of the *Gladiator's* crew began in earnest and an hour after the collision Captain Lumsden was brought ashore. The *St. Paul* then returned to Southampton where she went into dock for extensive repairs.

Attention now turned to the fort which was full of exhausted and injured seamen dressed in royal blue and khaki. Some of the badly injured were sent off to Golden Hill Fort Military Hospital. By the following day Lumsden could report the final death toll to Portsmouth, one lieutenant and 28 men, most of them drowned and swept away by the tide.

The *Gladiator* presented a big problem for her salvors as she lay on her damaged side. It took a total of five months to strip the ship of her armament and block off all her outlets for pumping, righting and raising the hull. It cost a small fortune, £50,000, but at the end of the day the ship was useless and was sold to a shipbreaker for £15,125.

There is one final peculiar twist to this tragic tale. Exactly ten years after the collision, on April 25th, 1918, the *St. Paul* unaccountably capsized and sank while at anchor in New York Harbour. The mystery of her loss was never resolved.

The Last Years of Peace 1908-1914

Between the loss of the *Gladiator* and the outbreak of the Great War there were a number of minor shipwrecks but no human casualties.

Of the notable wrecks the greatest waste was the brand new Belgian steam trawler *Nemrod*. On the night of February 6th, 1910, the *Nemrod* was lost in a thick fog and found an unexpected berth just under Walpen Chine. She ran straight up the beach and alerted the locality with continual blasts of her siren. Four members of the Wheeler family and the lifeboat's Second Coxswain scrambled down to the beach and at some risk rescued four of the crew. One knew a few words of English and kept repeating "Six in a boat." Fearing that they might attempt to land the boat in the dangerous groundswell, the rescuers alerted and launched the lifeboat. The new Atherfield boat *Gem* failed to find the *Nemrod's* boat which rowed around to Wheelers Bay, just past Ventnor. There they were rescued by more Wheelers, cousins of those at Blackgang.

Although the crew were all saved their fine ship was too close inshore to be salvaged. She quickly swung broadside onto the beach and heeled over on her side, littering the beach with her cargo of 70 tons of fish. The shore was soon busy with locals making sure that none of it went to waste. There was a good variety, "cod, haddock, gurnet, plaice, sole and turbot, and beauties they were too."

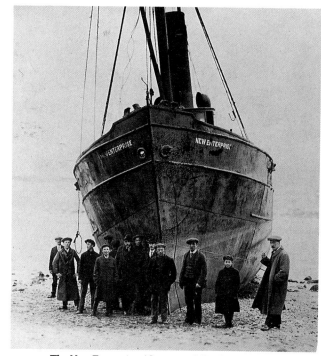

The New Enterprise. (Courtesy of Gordon Phillips).

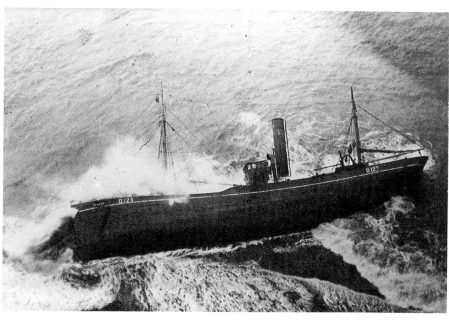

The Nemrod.

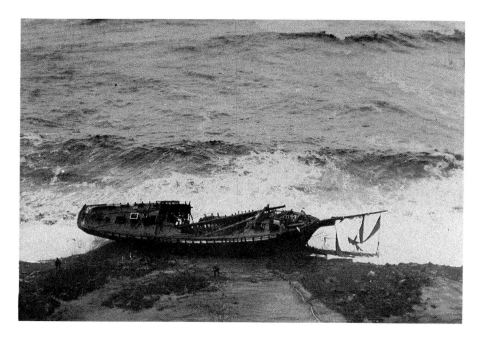

This is the schooner Prim, stranded, dismasted and beaten to a shambles by the sea. Sudmore Point, February 22nd, 1912. (Courtesy of Dave Wheeler).

The shore was also scattered with baskets from the ship to make collecting the fish easier. However, despite this bonanza the locals still felt sad that such a new ship should be left to the sea. "It seemed a sin to see such a clean smart looking craft bashed to pieces." The *Nemrod* was eventually blown apart with dynamite.

French Ketch Lost at Watcombe

Later on in the year on November 27th, a French ketch, *Rene,* was broken on the rocks in Watcombe Bay. Earlier that night she had grounded at Sudmore Point. The Brook boat *Susan Ashley* was launched to her aid but the *Rene* refloated and disappeared into the black night, heading west. A few hours later she came to rest at Watcombe, just west of Freshwater Bay, still under full sail. The crew of four took to their boat and steered for the small beach. Their boat was capsized by the groundswell but they all managed to stagger out of the surf. The *Rene* was less lucky. She split up on the rocks, losing her valuable cargo of zinc ore.

The New Enterprise

In 1913 another steam trawler came ashore, the *New Enterprise*. She was stranded on the soft beach of Sandown Bay and was salvaged and sold to the Turkish government. She served with the Turkish navy until she was sunk by the British during the Gallipoli campaign in 1915.

The Great War, 1914-1918

In the first week of August, 1914, a century of European peace and progress came to an abrupt end in four years of carnage, the Great War. At first the waters of the Wight were not affected. The great German fleet was bottled up; but later in the war German submarines sank a huge number of merchant ships in the Channel south of the Island.

The first effect of the outbreak of hostilities was the weakening of the Island's rescue services as the coastguards were immediately drafted and many lifeboatmen volunteered. When the Newcastle schooner *Theodora* came ashore on Bembridge Ledge on March 19th, 1915, the weakened lifeboat crew and launchers were unable to launch the boat. It was thrown broadside onto the rocks and two of the crew and one of the launchers were carried away from the scene suffering from exhaustion. Despite being drenched and frozen in the breaking surf the rest managed to launch the *Queen Victoria* and proceeded to the schooner which was not in great danger and was later towed back into deep water.

The following February the *Queen Victoria* was called out to a far more serious wreck; the paddle steamer *Empress Queen,* an Isle of Man ferry being used as a troopship. On February 3rd, 1916, she went aground on the Ring Rocks off Bembridge with over 100 men on board. The *Queen Victoria* made a series of dangerous and difficult trips to the stricken ferry. On the third journey the lifeboat was driven out of control and crashed onto the rocks of the ledge, suffering some damage. Nonetheless the crew relaunched her and made a fourth round trip to the *Empress Queen,* saving in all 110 men, a cat and a dog. Coxswain John Holbrook was awarded the R.N.L.I. Silver Medal. The masts of the *Empress Queen* can still be seen poking through the water at low tide.

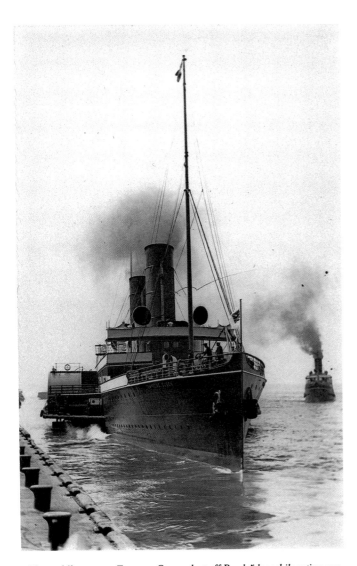

The paddle steamer Empress Queen, lost off Bembridge while acting as a troopship in February, 1916. (Courtesy of Tom Rayner).

Dramatic Rescue on Brook Ledge

The following night the Norwegian barque *Souvenir* was driven ashore at Brook. The soldiers guarding the coast did not understand her desperate signals and it was not until the next morning that the Brook lifeboat *Susan Ashley* was launched to the rescue. Great seas crashed over the lifeboat, driving her back towards the shore, and it proved impossible to close on the battered wreck of the barque. The 10 crew of the *Souvenir* could hear their ship tearing apart on the rocks below and one by one they leapt into the boiling surf and swam for the *Susan Ashley;* all except the Captain who stuck with his ship. The lifeboat picked up all nine swimmers but the ship's steward died as he lay in the bottom of the boat. Once the lifeboat was safely ashore the drenched and exhausted survivors were hauled out. The Captain was washed in with the pulped and smashed remains of the ship shortly after the lifeboat returned ashore. Coxswain Ben Jacobs received the Silver Medal thanks to this excellent and timely rescue.

The Loss of the Mendi: 650 Drowned

The greatest local human disaster of the war was the loss of *R.M.S. Mendi,* a steamer on the Cape-West Africa-Liverpool run that was bringing 800 black South African labourers to work behind the trenches in France.

At 5 a.m. on February 20th, 1917, she was steaming with a destroyer as escort 12 miles from St. Catherine's. There was a dense fog and without warning the bow of the liner *Darro* loomed out of the darkness and smashed into the *Mendi's* starboard side. Lacking the time to launch her boats she keeled over and sank in 20 minutes, throwing the crew and labourers into the icy black sea. The fog and darkness hindered the rescue and no less than 650 men perished in the intense cold.

Unrestricted Submarine Warfare

Through 1916 German submarines took a heavy toll of Allied shipping. In January, 1917, they began "unrestricted submarine warfare" sinking ships of all nations without warning around Britain's shores. It was a desperate gamble as it brought America into the war but it nearly succeeded; British shipping losses trebled in 1917. Eight ships were destroyed in a 30 mile radius of the Island in May, including the *S.S. Camberwell,* mined just six miles east-south-east of Dunnose Point on May 18th with the loss of seven lives. In October the 2,123 ton *S.S. Redesmere* was torpedoed three miles off St. Catherine's with the loss of 19 lives. In December another five ships were sunk; 15 men died and 10,000 tons of shipping went to the bottom.

Six more ships were destroyed around the Island in January, 1918, totalling 22,635 tons of shipping. The greatest of these was the 9,044 ton armed merchant escort ship *Mechanician.* On January 20th, two torpedoes ripped open her 500 foot hull. Her crew was able to beach her on the western side of the Shingles where she sank into a shallow grave and was soon buried in the shoal. This huge ship was never relocated. Two days later the torpedoed 3,677 ton armed merchantman *Serrana* limped as far as the Needles Bridge before she broke in two and foundered. In February another five ships were lost. 34 men went down with the 2,000 ton *Eleanor* nine miles off St. Catherine's and 20 more perished with the 5,000 ton *Huntsmoor.*

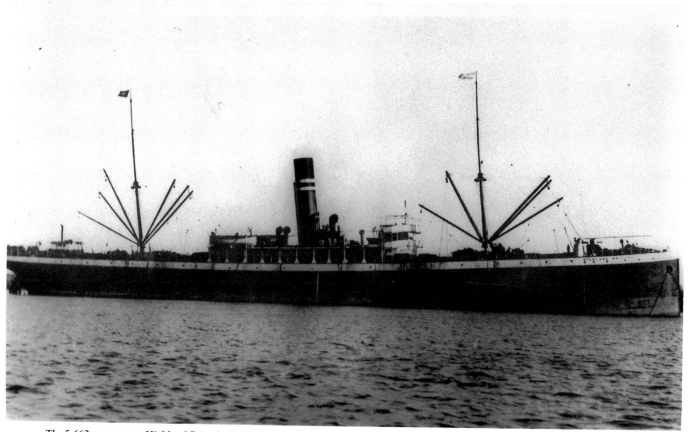

The 5,662 ton steamer Highland Brigade, built at Glasgow in 1901, she was torpedoed south-east of St. Catherine's Point on April 7th, 1918. She limped on to a point eight miles south by east of Shanklin pier where she foundered.

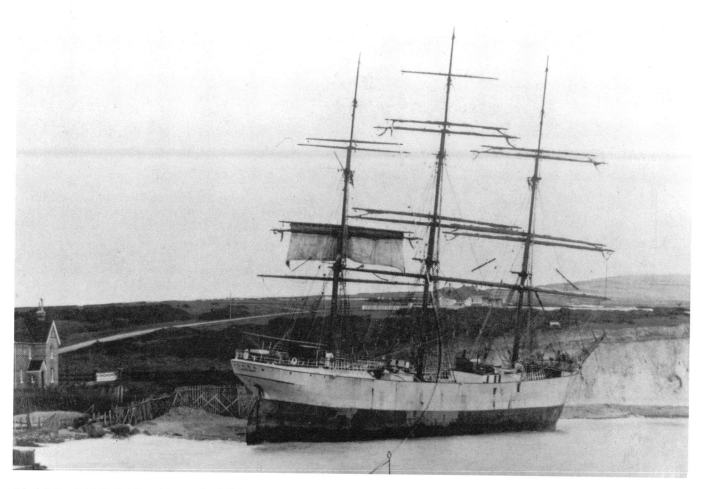

The full rigged ship Carl, driven right over the chalk bar and onto the cliff of Freshwater Bay on November 4th, 1916, by strong winds and a high tide. The crew were able to come ashore by scrambling up the bowsprit and into a garden. After a passage had been dynamited through the chalk bar, the Carl was safely rescued from her perilous berth. (Courtesy of Tom Rayner).

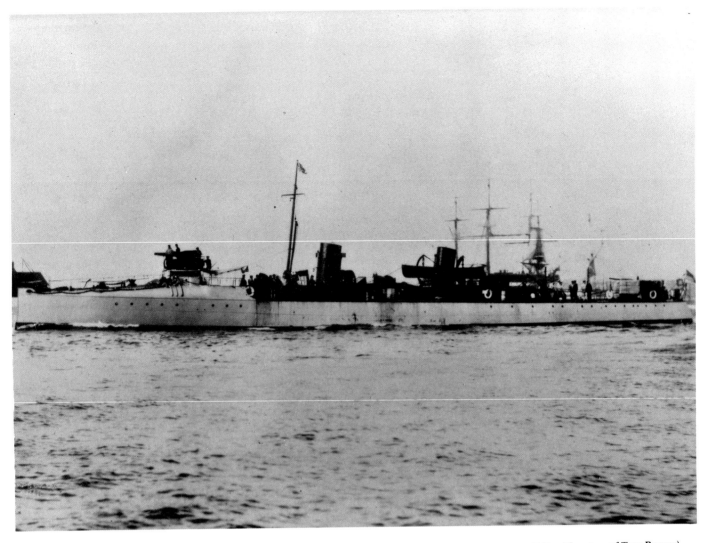

The torpedo boat destroyer Boxer, built at Cowes in the mid 1890's and sunk off Bembridge after a collision in February, 1918. (Courtesy of Tom Rayner).
Another torpedo boat destroyer, H.M.S. Velox, was lost in 1915 when it was mined off the Nab Light Vessel on October 25th.

'The Bacon and Lard Special'

One of the most memorable local wrecks was the large British tramp steamer *War Knight*. On March 24th she collided with the American tanker *O. B. Jennings* while they were proceeding up Channel in a large convoy. The tanker was carrying naptha and ignited in a massive explosion, killing almost everyone aboard the two ships.

The two burning vessels were towed towards the Island by two destroyers. The *O. B. Jennings* burned for 10 days in Sandown Bay and was then torpedoed. She was later repaired and refloated only to be torpedoed by a 'U' boat in the Atlantic a few months later. The unfortunate *War Knight* struck a mine and was finally sunk by gunfire in shallow water just off Watcombe Bay. This stopped the fire but the steamer's hull split open spilling out her cargo of bacon, lard, flour, oil and rubber. The people of Freshwater, tightly rationed, could hardly believe their luck. Crowds of people rushed to the shore opposite the blackened remains of the ship "arriving in carts and horse drawn wagons, some pushing prams and others wheeling bicycles, any type of vehicle to carry away sides of bacon and 28 lb. boxes of lard." Fred Mew was stationed nearby and was soon on the scene "What a sight met my eyes, parts of pigs going in all directions. For many weeks the Bay was a scene of great activity, huge stacks of salvaged cargo reaching from end to end."

Once the authorities had re-established control, 38 people were arrested and summoned to Newport by rail. Their train was locally dubbed "the Bacon and Lard Special."

Another ship sunk just off the Island was the 4,284 ton *S.S. Luis*. On April 12th, 1918, this two year old steamer was carrying cased oil, flour and artillery shells to France when she was torpedoed 3½ miles off St. Catherine's; four of the crew were killed in the explosion. She was taken in tow for Sandown Bay, but foundered in 32 feet of water just off Luccombe Chine.

On April 30th the 2,871 ton *S.S. Isleworth* was sunk only three miles south-west of Ventnor Pier with the loss of 29 lives, but after that only two more ships were destroyed in local waters before the German submarines abandoned the Channel for good.

Defeat of the 'U' Boats

From March onwards the losses of Allied shipping began to fall off as more 'U' boats were destroyed by mines and surface ships. The Dover Straights were blocked with nets and minefields forcing the submarines to use the long northern route around Scotland. While the Allied blockade of Germany bit home, starving the people and closing the factories, American troops and supplies poured into France, unhindered by 'U' boat attacks.

On October 25th the last remaining 'U' boats were recalled to cover a final suicide voyage by the German battlefleet. Nine days later the German navy mutinied, sparking the revolution that ended the Great War on November 11th, 1918.

In its attempted blockade of Britain the German navy sank over 50 large ships in a 30 mile radius of the Island, totalling 132,000 tons of shipping. However it was the Royal Navy that again proved its mastery of the seas and it was the British blockade which finally starved the German people into submission. The numerous wrecks around the Island are now happy hunting grounds for aqualung divers, both archaeologists and amateur souvenir hunters. This is an attractive past-time but beware of the cargoes, explosives become highly unstable under water.

The Interwar Years: 1919-1939

The twenties and thirties saw few shipwrecks on the Island. In the economic shadow of the Great War, with so much of the world's wealth destroyed, and in a time of bitter trade wars, shipping almost disappeared. While the ports were filled with rusting hulks, the seas were almost empty.

There was a brief trade revival in 1919. That year saw two American shipwrecks on Bembridge Ledge, the troopship *Narracansett* and the *S.S. Wakulla,* which came ashore on an August night in a strong southerly gale and a heavy sea. The lifeboat *Queen Victoria* saved all 13 crew. The coxswain, John Holbrook, received a second Service Clasp to his Silver Medal.

Only four big ships came ashore between 1920 and 1939. The first of these was the steam trawler *Lois,* which came ashore in a thick fog in June, 1921. Fred Mew heard two ships go ashore and slid down the cliff on the seat of his trousers to find the Fleetwood trawler *Lois* hard aground, "her bows high and dry on the shingle." Mew shouted to the men aboard and then re-ascended the cliff to alert the rocket crew. The other ship had grounded on Hawk Ledge, but she refloated in the night. The crew of the *Lois* were taken off by motor boat. The trawler was hauled off the beach of Chale Bay after extensive salvage work but she grounded on a sandbank just 50 yards out and was abandoned to the sea.

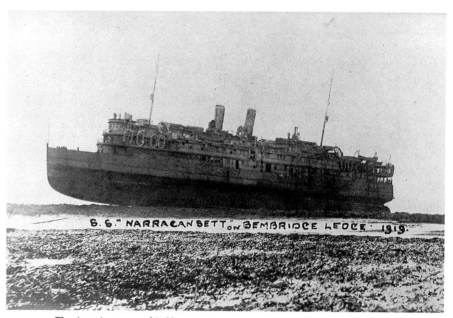

The American troopship Narracansett stranded on Bembridge Ledge in 1919. (Courtesy of Beken of Cowes).

The next wreck on the Back of the Wight was the 216 ton motor trading vessel *Capable.* She left Poole Harbour on the night of March 3rd, 1930, and soon became hopelessly lost in a blinding fog. At 10.30 her hull bashed heavily against an outcrop of the Atherfield Ledge, the engines were put out of action and the crippled vessel was driven closer inshore by the big Atlantic swell. The coastguard alerted the Yarmouth Lifeboat, *B.A.S.P.* and the Blackgang Life Saving Apparatus crew. As the *B.A.S.P.* was passing Brook Coxswain Walter Cotton noted some flares and steered inshore to investigate. As he did so, the lifeboat was picked up by the ocean swell and thrown against one of the slimy protrusions of Brook Ledge, where she remained hard aground. The flares Cotton had seen were the launching signal of the Brook lifeboat *Susan Ashley.* She was rowed straight to Atherfield but arrived to find that the crew of the *Capable* had been rescued by the Blackgang L.S.A. volunteers, who were all completely drenched by the swell but were given dry clothes and hot drinks by the coastguards.

It took another four days to refloat the Yarmouth lifeboat which was only achieved with the help of a number of engineers from Cowes shipyards and 150 troops from Parkhurst Barracks. The *Capable* was also saved and towed to Southampton, one of the few ships to escape the grip of Atherfield Ledge.

The Roumelian

Two years later on May 5th, 1932, the 2,600 ton steamer *Roumelian* collided with the *S.S. St. Nazare* 24 miles south-west of the Needles. The lightly damaged *St. Nazare* continued her journey while the *Roumelian* limped towards the safety of the Solent. She had 56 crew and passengers on board and was taking in water fast; so her Captain radioed to the Island for assistance. The Sunday evening service at Brook church was interrupted and abandoned and the *Susan Ashley* quickly launched. Lord Mottistone, a proud member of the crew, recorded that the unwieldy lifeboat covered 4½ miles in just 40 minutes. Nevertheless it was clear that the days of the rowing lifeboat were over as the Yarmouth lifeboat *B.A.S.P.* roared across the sea to rendezvous with the stricken steamer five miles south-west of the Needles, picking up the pilot on the way. The *Susan Ashley* returned to station while the *B.A.S.P.* put the pilot aboard the *Roumelian,* took off four passengers, and lead the crippled ship through the Needles Channel.

Just past Yarmouth the steamer's pumps conceded defeat and the *Roumelian* sank in the shallow waters of Hampstead Ledge. After a difficult salvage in which two of the crew died in an accident, the *Roumelian* was refloated and taken to London for repairs.

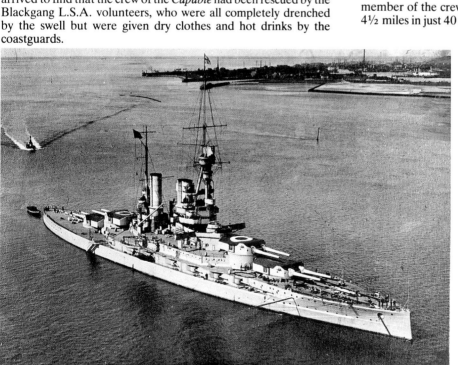

The German Imperial Battlecruiser S.M.S. Baden. Surrendered to the British at the end of the war, she was used as a target for testing British shells against her Krupp armour and was then ignominiously scuttled in St. Catherine's Deep on August 16th, 1921. (Courtesy of the Imperial War Museum).

The Luigi Accame

The last big wreck before the war was the 5,000 ton Italian steamer *Luigi Accame*. Based at Genoa, the ship was bound from Algeria to Rotterdam with a cargo of iron ore. On April 6th, 1937, her siren was heard wailing in a thick fog close to Rocken End. The coastguards fired warning rockets but to no avail. The Italian steamer ploughed onto the rocks three quarters of a mile west of St. Catherine's Lighthouse. At 10 p.m. the new Yarmouth lifeboat, *S.G.E.*, motored out of the harbour into the dense fog. The Blackgang L.S.A. team were called out too but they could not get a line to the ship which was 400 yards offshore.

At 12.30 the lifeboat reached the *Luigi Accame,* picking up the 29 crew in two lifeboats drifting to seaward of the ship. "There was a heavy groundswell at the time" recalls Geoff Cotton, one of *S.G.E.'s* crew, "and we could hear the steamers steel plates tearing as she moved in the swell." The Italians boarded the lifeboat and their boats were taken in tow, arriving at Yarmouth at 5.15 a.m.

It was the end of May before the *Luigi Accame* was sufficiently patched up to refloat her and tow her to Southampton, and during this time she took a regular beating from the sea. According to Geoff Cotton she was "fit only for scrap when they got her into dock, her bottom having been torn to shreds." Despite this she was repaired and sold to a Dutch company, only to be sunk by a German armed merchantman during the Second World War.

A few days after the wreck of the *Luigi Accame,* on April 15th, the Brook lifeboat *Susan Ashley* was launched a final time and rowed to Yarmouth where she was later sold. The Brook station was closed, bringing to an end the heroic era of the rowing lifeboats. During the 77 years of service the three lifeboats of the south-west coast had saved a total of 826 lives.

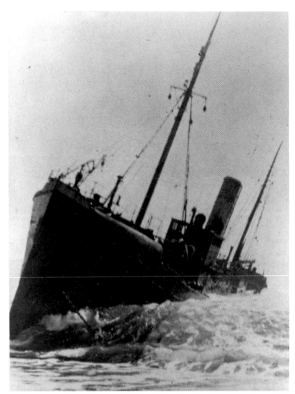

The steam trawler Lois, ashore in Chale Bay in June, 1921. Despite salvage operations she was a total loss.

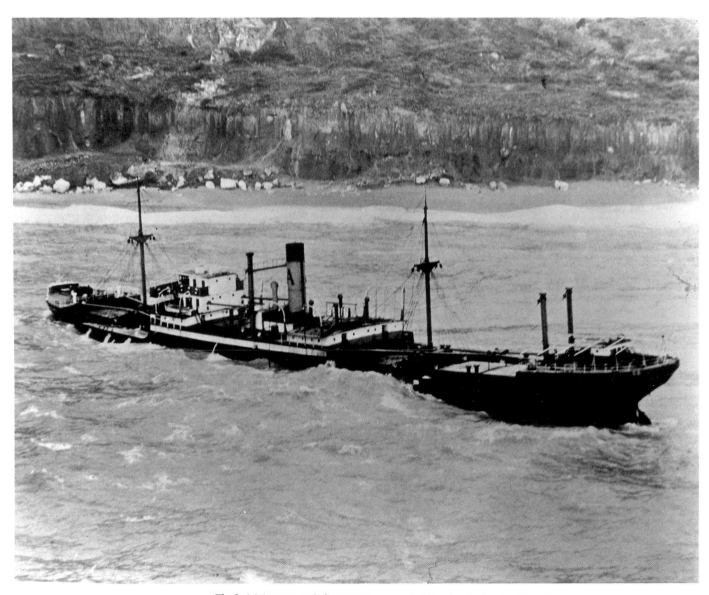

The Luigi Accame, an Italian steamer aground off Rocken End in April, 1937.

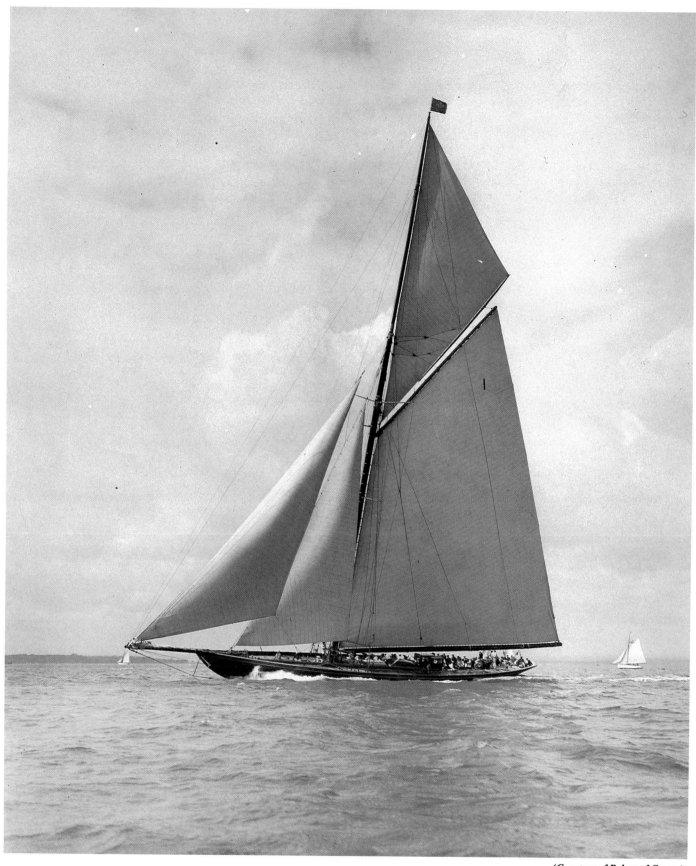

(Courtesy of Beken of Cowes)

The Britannia

One of the most famous vessels sunk off the Island is the royal cutter *Britannia* which lies somewhere off St. Catherine's. The *Britannia* was the inspiration and flagship of the British yachting world for over 40 years. Completed in 1893 for Prince Edward, she had a strong but light hull 121 feet long with lines so perfect that 30 years later alterations of only one twentieth of an inch could be suggested. Her sail spread 172 feet from the tip of her bowsprit to the end of her 92 feet boom, and reached up 142 feet to the tip of her mast. She had seven different rigs in her long life, going from the 10,000 square feet of her original gaff rig to her final 8,337 foot Bermudan rig of 1935. She had an extraordinary career, reviving

first class yacht racing in the 1890's and the 1920's. In all she took part in 634 races of which she won 231 and came second or third in another 129. Only in the 1930's did she begin to fade. In 1935 she entered 20 races but won no prizes. Her owner, George V, still enjoyed the season. He was a great sportsman and deeply attached to the *Britannia*. When he died in January, 1936, it was decided that the old yacht should follow him to the grave. She was stripped down and her hull towed away from her Cowes berth by the navy on the bright morning of July 9th, watched by a small group of her devotees including Uffa Fox. She was towed to the south of the Island and then sunk by detonating an explosive charge in her hull.

The Second World War: 1939-1945

On September 3rd, 1939, Britain declared war on Nazi Germany and entered into a six year struggle that nearly led to the complete defeat of the British Empire. The Island and the waters around it became the country's front line of defence in 1940, and later became one of the launching points for the invasion of Normandy in 1944. Thankfully, few ships came ashore in the traditional way at a time when sea rescue services were highly restricted. The lighthouses were shut down and ships sailed without lights to avoid enemy attacks. Minefields were laid all around the Island. The Bembridge lifeboat could not launch without warning the artillery battery on Culver Down. The crew were issued with two rifles in case of contact with the Germans. The lifeboats also suffered from their crews being conscripted, and took a back seat to the navy escort ships which did almost all the offshore rescue work.

The Naval Trawler Britisher

One of the few ships ashore during the war was the naval trawler *H.M.S. Britisher,* which was wrecked on the foul night of November 14th, 1939. The trawler was driven ashore on Brighstone Ledge in "a gale of wind, pouring rain and a darkness that could be felt." Both the Yarmouth lifeboat and the Blackgang L.S.A. company had great difficulty in reaching the ship. The rocket company found the Military Road blocked with troops and when they finally arrived opposite the battered trawler, the wide waterlogged clay cliffs barred them from the beach.

The Yarmouth lifeboat *S.G.E.,* under Coxswain Walter Cotton, struggled out through the Needles Channel in complete darkness and pitched and rolled in the swell down to Brighstone. Just as she approached the wreck one of the crew collapsed. He needed medical attention immediately. After considering the tide, Cotton made a difficult decision and the *S.G.E.* turned away from the *Britisher* and began to fight her way back to the Solent.

The burden of rescue now fell on the rocket crew. The *Britisher* presented a poor target, being 300 yards out and end on to the shore. Great seas were breaking over the ship which could barely be seen through the thick rain. The first rocket went across the ship but was carried away by the wind. As the rocket lines became wetter and heavier each one fell short until the Blackgang men signalled to the ship asking the crew to float a line ashore. On their second attempt the beleagured crew succeeded. The problem now was to collect the line. "There was no path to the shore, the cliffs were just sheer running clay . . . With great difficulty the cliff ladders were rolled down, but they stuck in the mud, and it seemed hopeless." At this point two men volunteered to descend the cliff. "Sometimes on top of the ladder, sometimes under it, covered in mud and drenched with rain they reached the shore."

Thanks to their courage the bosun's chair was set up and two men were hauled to safety. At this point the little *S.G.E.* arrived back on the scene.

After another perilous journey through the blackened western Solent, Cotton had left his unconscious crewman aboard the *Star of India* and then returned immediately to Brighstone. As the trawler was in shallow water the only way the lifeboat could safely approach it was by anchoring and veering down on her. Once the anchor slipped, and each time she came in her hull bounced on the ledge below. Six times she swung past the wreck, allowing all 12 of the remaining crew to leap into her. The *S.G.E.* arrived back at Yarmouth at 10.30 a.m. Walter Cotton was later awarded the Bronze Medal by the R.N.L.I. The Bembridge coxswain Harry Gawn, was also awarded a Bronze Medal following the rescue of the 21 crew of the naval minesweeper *H.M.S. Kingston Cairngorm.*

1940: The Brink of Defeat

After eight months of stalemate on the Western Front the German offensive of May, 1940 encircled, killed and captured a million Allied troops in a month and a month later France was overrun. Only the Channel now stood between the Nazi armies and the English coast. The Island and the surrounding sea came under repeated attacks from submarines, torpedo boats and waves of bombers, dive bombers and fighters.

Among the casualties of this time was the 216 ton motor vessel *Capable* which previously went ashore at Atherfield in 1930. She was blown apart by a mine just outside the Spithead on June 5th, 1940. On June 22nd, the anti-submarine yacht *Campeador 5* suffered a similar end, and on July 24th, the 2,318 ton *S.S. Terlings* was sunk by German aircraft 10 miles south-west of St. Catherine's.

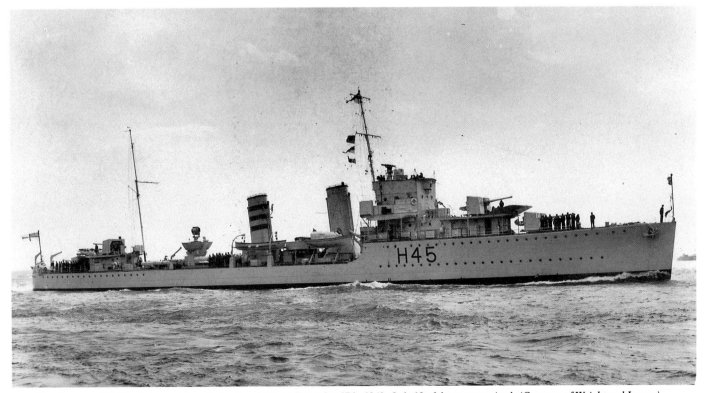

The destroyer H.M.S. Acheron, blown in two by a mine on December 17th, 1940. Only 13 of the crew survived. (Courtesy of Wright and Logan).

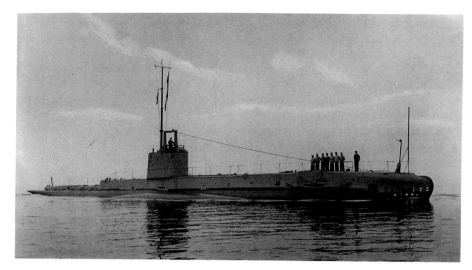

The 'S' Class submarine Swordfish, blown apart by a mine south of St. Catherine's on November 7th, 1940. All 40 crew perished. (Courtesy of Wright and Logan).

Convoy Attacked: Three Sunk

Britain's greatest defeat in Island waters came on August 8th, 1940,when the Luftwaffe launched a series of attacks on a British convoy about 15 miles south-west of St. Catherines's. Despite the fierce anti-aircraft fire of the convoy's escorts and the guns aboard the merchantmen, the German planes dived through the clouds of flak to score a series of direct hits. The 1,597 ton *Coquetdale* and the 942 ton Dutch steamer *Ajax* both erupted in smoke and flame and crash dived the Channel floor where the two ships still lie in a communal tangle of wreckage, 112 feet down. A few hours later the Luftwaffe completed the day's work by sinking the 1,042 ton *Empire Crusader,* a few miles to the north.

German Mines Sink Two Naval Ships

Through the Autumn of 1940 the R.A.F. held off the German air attacks and the Nazi invasion plans were called off. However, the British continued to suffer damaging losses.

Among them was the submarine *H.M.S. Swordfish.* She left Portsmouth on November 7th, bound for a station off the German naval base at Brest, and was never heard of again. It was assumed that she had been sunk by German destroyers off Brittany but in 1983 marine archaeologist and diver Martin Woodward, of Bembridge Maritime Museum, discovered the submarine in two

parts, south of St. Catherine's. It appears that the *Swordfish* met her unexpected end just a few hours after leaving base. As she dived for the first time she was blown apart by a powerful mine. Woodward found the escape hatch open but concluded that even if some of the 40 crew had made their escape, they stood no chance in the cold November seas, far from land.

Just over a month later the 1,775 ton destroyer *Acheron* set off for high speed trials south of the Island with a full complement of 190 men and 25 dockyard officials. It was the early morning of December 17th, a bitterly cold night made worse by a raw north-easterly wind. "It was an awful winter and there was ice on the shores" recalls one of the ship's stokers, Reg Willis.

Just before 7 a.m. the *Acheron* was turning to make her eastward run when she struck a German mine. "There was a muffled roar and the darkness was transformed to brilliant light as she erupted in flame." The destroyer was blown in two. When Reg Willis reached the top of the escape hatch, "I saw the bow was missing. I just jumped, there was nothing else to do." Most of the 215 men aboard went down with the ship which sank in minutes. The survivors clung to Carley floats and pieces of wreckage but because of the intense cold of that freezing early morning only 19 men were picked up alive some hours later.

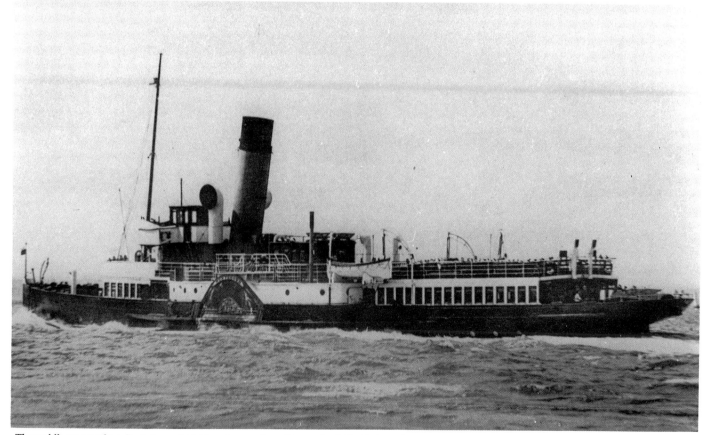

The paddle steamer ferry Portsdown. At 4.30 on the morning of September 20th, 1941, the 342 ton Portsdown was steaming from Portsmouth to Ryde when she was blown up and sunk by a mine. (Courtesy of Tom Rayner).

The Battle of the Atlantic 1941-1944

In 1941 Germany reverted to the Great War strategy of submarine blockade to starve Britain into surrender. The Royal Navy was unable to meet the threat of the 'U' boats and the British merchant fleet began to suffer appalling losses. By September, 1941, Britain's imports had been halved and had these losses continued the British people would have starved. The casualty rate among merchant seamen was horrific. Out of a total of 145,000 men, all volunteer civilians on wages of just £9 a month, no less than 32,000 died through enemy action.

Britain's position improved when the United States entered the war in 1941 but it was not until April, 1943, that the tide of the battle turned, when the British introduced the Centimetric Radar. In a month one third of all 'U' boats at sea had been destroyed and Germany was thrown onto the defensive.

The Allies Victorious, 1944-1945

In 1944 attention switched back to the Channel as Britain, the U.S.A. and Canada prepared huge forces for the invasion of France. The Germans were quite unable to stop the vast armada that carried the Allied forces to Normandy, or to cut the bustling lines of supply that fed the growing bridgehead. In the actual invasion one British 586 ton landing craft foundered off the Needles. A few days later on June 10th German torpedo boats sunk the 621 ton *S.S. Dungrange* and the 534 ton *M.V. Ashanti*, both about six miles south-west of St. Catherine's. Eight days later the 1,764 ton *S.S. Albert C. Field* was sent to the bottom about 20 miles south-west of the Needles, loaded with ammunition. On July 27th the 2,938 ton Belgian ex-cross Channel ferry *H.M.S. Prince Leopold*, then being used as an infantry landing ship, was torpedoed, capsized and sank about 13 miles east of Dunnose Point.

These losses had little effect on the Allied advance in France and by the end of the autumn all the German naval bases in France had been taken and the Channel had been cleared of the enemy.

The last incident of the war occurred on April 6th, 1945. The Commander of the German submarine *U1195* saw in his periscope the 11,420 ton passenger liner *S.S. Cuba* with an escort of six destroyers, moving grandly across Sandown Bay to pick up troops

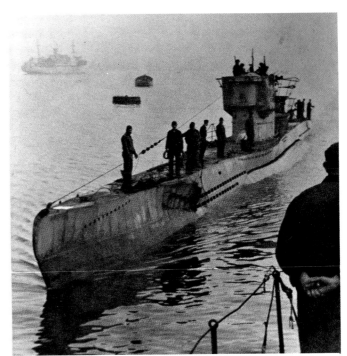

A Class 7C 'U' Boat of the same type as the U1195; destroyed in Sandown Bay after sinking the S.S. Cuba. (Courtesy of J.P. Mallmann-Showell).

at Portsmouth. In an act of suicidal bravery the 'U' boat torpedoed and sank the great ship about nine miles east of Dunnose Point. The destroyers then mercilessly hunted down the German submarine which got to about 12 miles south by east of Sandown. There she settled on the seabed 25 metres down and shut down her generators to foil the destroyers detection equipment. It was to no avail. The six destroyers pounded the seabed with their powerful depth charges until one from *H.M.S. Watchman* came close enough to blow the submarine apart. This was the last local wreck of the war. In the first few days of May, 1945, Berlin was conquered and the war came to an end.

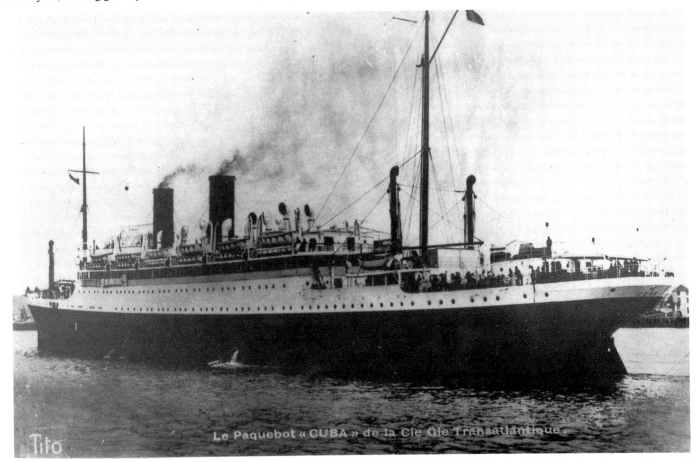

The 11,420 ton passenger liner S.S. Cuba, sunk by a 'U' boat on the edge of Sandown Bay on April 5th, 1945. She was built in 1923 by Swan Hunters of Newcastle for the French Lines Service to the West Indies and Central America. The submarine which sank her was destroyed in the same action.

(Courtesy of Tom Rayner).

The Post War Years

The post war era saw an immediate revival of commerce and therefore of shipping, but the number of shipwrecks remained thankfully low and declined as time went by. The comprehensive system of navigation buoys, pilot services, lighthouses and lightships operated by Trinity House, and the growing sophistication of navigational instruments all made shipwrecks much more unlikely. Nevertheless, the traditional hazards of the Island's coasts were still able to bring down disaster on the unlucky or careless mariner.

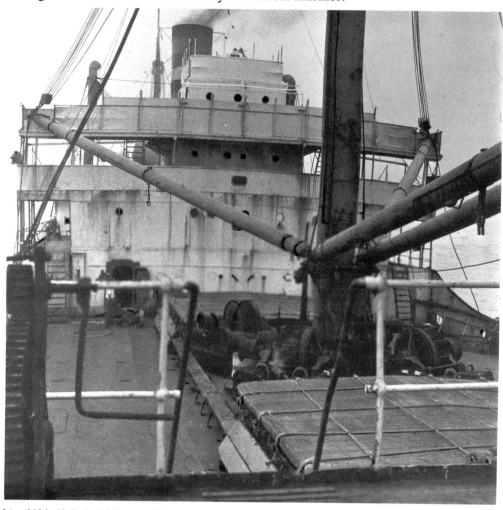

In the early morning of April 15th, 1947, the 5,000 ton coal bearing S.S. Georgie drifted off course during a thick fog and crunched ashore on Rocken End, about 400 yards from the cliff. Her bows were badly damaged and she began to take in water, but given the size of the ship there was no danger to the crew. Tugs dragged her back into the sea just a few days later. (Courtesy of Viv Spencer).

Islay Mist : Cliff Rescue

Two of the most spectacular wrecks of the late forties were pleasure boats driven ashore by stormy weather at Watcombe Bay and Binnel Bay. In both cases tragedy was only averted by the prompt action and characteristic bravery of the rescue services.

The first of these was the 50 ton motor launch *Islay Mist* which was driven towards the sheer chalk face of Freshwater's cliffs by a force 7 southerly gale, on the night of August 27th, 1947. There were three men, a woman and two children on board. Their vessel was driven onto the rocks beneath the 350 foot cliffs of Watcombe Bay.

When the Yarmouth lifeboat *S.G.E.* reached the scene it was impossible to get close to the wreck. She instead stood off and illuminated the scene with her searchlights. On top of the cliff the Freshwater Life Saving Apparatus team had set up their rocket, and at 4.15 a.m., they successfully fired a line across the beleaguered launch. This was hauled in by those on board with a cliff ladder attached to it. At daybreak two coastguards descended the unsteady ladder to the wreck below and brought up the occupants one at a time. It was still blowing a fresh gale and it must have been a hair raising experience for all concerned. The rescuers were honoured with a shield and Bronze Medals and the owner of the *Islay Mist* gave £100 to be shared among all those who had helped to save his life.

The Wreck of the Yacht Hope

On the morning of August 8th, 1948, the coastguards at Atherfield saw the auxiliary yacht *Hope* drifting across Chale Bay and showing distress signals. The weather was appalling. Throughout the night the sea had been driven eastward by a howling gale intensified by thick rain squalls, and morning brought no relief from the wind and rain. The coastguards telephoned Fred Mew, then head of Blackgang Life Saving Apparatus crew. As soon as enough men were gathered to carry the rocket gear, they set off along the coast following the damaged yacht as she struggled to stay off the rocks. As the rocket crew climbed through the mud and rocks of the overgrown undercliff the nine people aboard the yacht managed to cheat the rocks of their prize until they reached Binnel Point. Then the *Hope* went over on her side and went to pieces under the beating of the waves. Her occupants had just enough time to jump, fall or be washed off the *Hope* before she was "smashed to atoms." The rocket crew waded into the surf as they arrived. Three of them dived into the sea to rescue two women who could be seen floating face down, their clothes entangled in the rocks. All nine were saved.

The three men who saved the two women, Vic Salter, Jim Richards and J. Grist of Ryde, all received Bronze medals from the Royal Humane Society. In the New Year's Honours List of 1950/51 Fred Mew was awarded the British Empire Medal for services with the Coast Life Saving Corps.

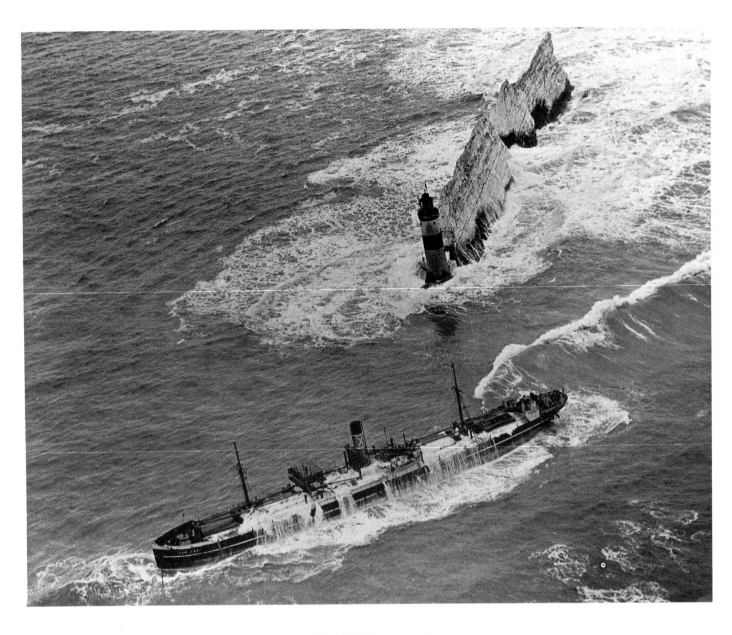

The S.S. Varvassi

On the clear morning of January 5th, 1947, the 3,874 ton Greek steamer *Varvassi* ploughed onto the Needles Bridge just 100 yards west-north-west of the Needles Lighthouse, where her rusted remains have stayed ever since.

The *Varvassi* was bound from Algiers to Southampton and Boulogne with a cargo of tangerines, wine and iron ore.

The cause of her grounding was something of a mystery. Captain Coufopandelis later claimed that the ship drifted out of control when he stopped her engines to pick up the pilot.

By midday the moderate south-easterly breeze had freshened to half a gale and there was a heavy swell running. With some difficulty Yarmouth boatbuilder Harry Simmonds put salvage officer Barker on board from his launch *Diane*. For three hours that afternoon the powerful Southampton tug *Calshot* struggled to anchor the ship. Twice the anchor chain broke in the swell but the task was finally accomplished.

At 7.15 Barker called out the Yarmouth lifeboat *S.G.E.* to stand by while the *Calshot* attempted to haul off the steamer at high water. The attempt had to be called off. The *Varvassi* was taking water and it was too dangerous to try and pull her off in the gathering storm and darkness. Huge seas smashed against the 32 year old plates of the rigid wreck and the lifeboatmen and tug crews were drenched by freezing rain and snow. The *Varvassi's* second engineer Vitsasakis won the praise of the rest of the crew by keeping up the steam pressure and thus maintaining the ship's straining pumps and electricity supply.

At 2.30 a.m. the lifeboat turned towards Yarmouth but the tired, lifeboatmen had hardly put their heads down when the maroons were fired again. Back at the Needles they found the *Varvassi* with great seas breaking right over her and threatening to wash the officers out of the bridge. The lifeboat had considerable difficulties in getting alongside. Several times the lines between the two vessels were broken by the violence of the sea. The huge seas crashing across the steamer's decks poured down onto the lifeboat. Nevertheless all 35 crew and the pilot officer and salvage officer were safely rescued.

At 1 o'clock that afternoon Simmonds took Coufopandelis and 12 volunteers back to the ship to rescue their personal belongings and pets, and to feed the seven heifers which were penned on the deck. They were being carried to provide fresh meat for the crew. It was two days before anyone could again board the stricken steamer. That morning Simmonds took a slaughterer to the ship to kill the wretched heifers and throw them overboard.

Repeated attempts were made to recover the *Varvassi*, but to no avail. The weather would not allow the salvors to get close to the ship for days on end. Her bottom was ripped open and she sank down into an early and shallow grave. Most of her cargo of tangerines was saved by local fishermen and sold ashore, a great treat for everyone after seven years of harsh rationing. Some large barrels of salty Algerian wine also washed ashore when the steamer broke up. Fred Mew thought it made "quite a good drink" when sweetened and heated. The ship itself broke up, remaining to this day as a hazard to shipping. Little of her now remains but some of her girders are still visible below the water at low tides.

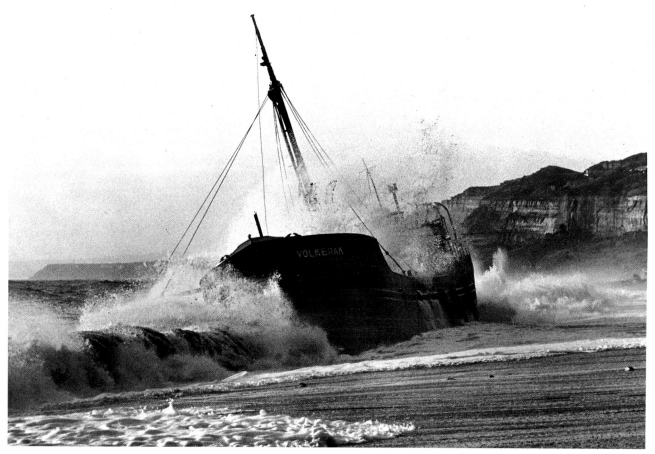

The Volkerak — a total wreck.

Bizarre Coincidence: The Volkerak and Albatross

In March, 1951 and December, 1952, two Dutch motor vessels, the *Volkerak* and the *Albatross* came ashore at the same spot. The 337 ton *Volkerak* was carrying china clay from Cornwall to Amsterdam when she lost her bearings in a thick fog, and was driven ashore by a strong gale a mile west of Rocken End. She was stranded broadside on to the sea, which smashed right over the ship with every wave. The Blackgang LSA crew had a terrible job reaching the ship across the chaos of slippery cliffs "just a mass of mud and every hole full of water." Nevertheless the apparatus was set up and fired and all eight men brought safely ashore. The *Volkerak* was a total loss.

Twenty-one months later the 83 ton *Albatross* lost her way in dense fog while bound from Penzance to Hull with a cargo of scrap. By an extraordinary stroke of bad luck she struck at the same spot as the gnarled remains of the *Volkerak,* whose iron mast greeted the newcomer by smashing through its hull. The three crew clambered ashore, one being injured and one losing his shoes, and made their way to the lighthouse where they were cared for by the keeper and his family until Fred Mew arrived to cater for them on behalf of the Shipwrecked Mariners Society. The *Albatross* was so badly damaged that only a little of her equipment was saved before she deteriorated into the same state as the *Volkerak.*

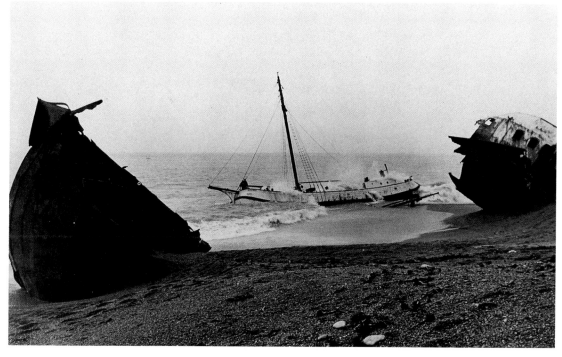

The Albatross, wrecked on the mast of the Volkerak.

The Virginia

One of the most dramatic rescues of the postwar era was that of the 21 crew of the *S.S. Virginia* brought ashore by breeches buoy at Atherfield on Christmas Eve, 1952.

The 2,041 ton steamer *Virginia* came ashore just two days after the *Albatross* and in similar conditions; thick fog, rain and heavy seas. The *Virginia* was registered in Panama but based at Alexandria. She was sailing from Bilboa to Bremen with a cargo of iron ore and a crew of 23 under Captain Galatis. At just before midnight on December 23rd, her forward steel plates buckled and screeched along the waiting rocks of Atherfield Ledge, 600 yards from the shore.

The coastguards alerted the Blackgang L.S.A. crew and the Yarmouth lifeboat, but that was recalled when Galatis radioed that his ship was in good condition and only required tugs. This did not deter Fred Mew's team who were soon manhandling their equipment through Atherfield Holiday Camp to set up the rocket apparatus on a slippery plateau 120 feet above the sea. Their first rocket splashed down into the waves. The wreck was too far away and the Blackgang men could hardly see it until the coastguards set up a searchlight at 1 a.m.

The weather steadily deteriorated until 3 a.m. when the *Virginia* began to signal repeatedly for tugs and a lifeboat. On the radio she reported that the ship's 35 year old plates were being smashed against the surrounding rocks by the sea, with No. 4 hold leaking badly. Then the rising sea pushed the steamer's protesting hull over the outer reef and drove her another 400 yards inshore. By 4.30 No. 3 and No. 4 holds and the engine room were flooded, and the radio short-circuited.

Matters began to improve after the tide peaked at 4.30 a.m. The Yarmouth lifeboat *S.G.E.* arrived at 5.10 a.m., and stood by for five hours, eventually taking off only two of the crew and all the crew's luggage. The rest decided to stay on, but as the wind freshened into a strong gale they changed their minds. A rocket line was fired to the ship and Mr. R. Dabell of Blackgang Chine went out to the ship to instruct the crew in the handling of the breeches buoy. The first of the *Virginia's* crew was hauled ashore at 1.30 and the rest came in a steady flow through the afternoon, the officers last. When Mr. Dabell returned ashore he brought a present of six bottles of brandy and 500 cigars from Captain Galatis for the rest of the rocket crew who had been on duty for over 12 hours and were drenched and caked in mud. A coastguard officer saw the first bottle disappearing and confiscated the rest as contraband. The rocket crew were livid, but matters were put right, as the County Press reported "... true to past traditions along this coast, the articles disappeared while the officer's back was momentarily turned."

The rescue was a great success. The entire ship's complement of 23 had been saved without injury. "I wish to give the greatest credit to my crew" wrote Fred Mew, "who throughout the long tiring day never faltered; in fact for some reason after the brandy came, and went, they seemed more cheery than ever."

Aided by unusually fine weather the *Virginia* was offloaded of 1,000 tons of ore, refloated a month later after a massive effort, and towed to Southampton for repairs.

The Kingsbridge

In the early hours of January 21st, 1955, the 7,142 ton freighter *Kingsbridge* stranded herself on Brighstone Ledge, 450 yards from the shore. The Blackgang L.S.A. crew set up their gear in the grounds of Brighstone Holiday Camp and awaited developments. By 3.30 p.m. the ship had been driven further in, and was battered and taking water. Her master requested a line. The 75 year old Fred Mew fired the rocket with precision accuracy, "just in front of her bridge, one of the ship's crew jumping hurriedly out of the way to the amusement of the large crowd on the cliff."

The Blackgang crew remained on call for a whole week as various attempts to refloat the ship were tried and failed. On Jaunary 28th the *Kingsbridge* was finally hauled back into the sea thanks to the combined efforts of Totland salvor V. Stallard, a helicopter, several tugs and the ship's own engines.

Later that year Fred Mew retired to Nettlestone after 50 years service in the lifeboat and rocket crews.

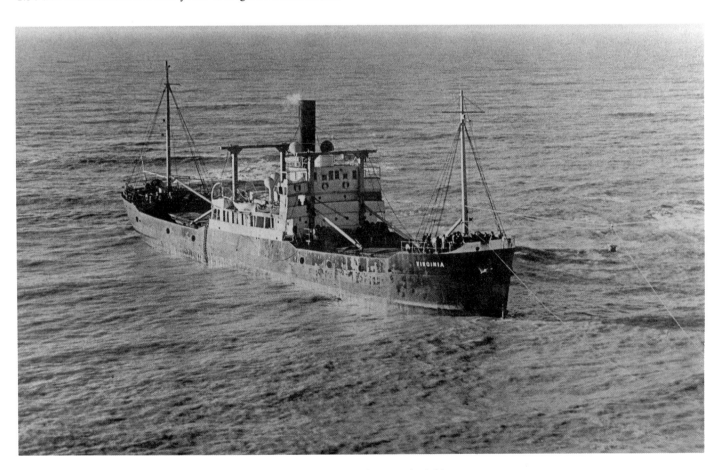

The S.S. Virginia ashore at Atherfield.

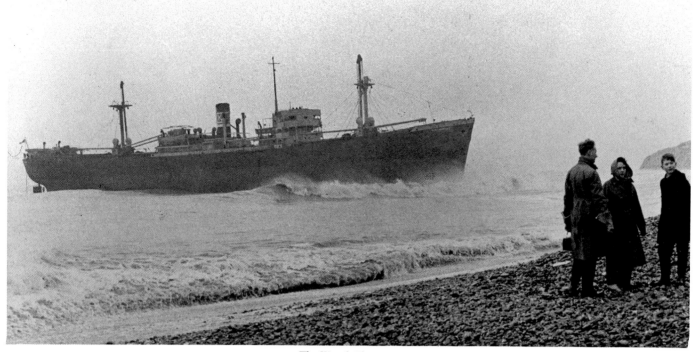

The Kingsbridge

The Iano

On November 4th, 1957, the 2,500 ton Italian steamer *Iano* took shelter from a storm in Sandown Bay. Her anchors slipped and she was driven broadside onto the beach between Sandown and Culver Cliff, only 150 yards from the shore. The Sandown L.S.A. company failed to get a line to the ship due to the strong wind and called out Ventnor L.S.A. team who fired a line to the ship in the early hours of the morning. The crew connected it to one of their lifeboats and in three trips landed 26 of the 30 crew.

These drenched and dishevelled Italians were taken to Shanklin Police Station, where they were reclothed and fed by Fred Mew on behalf of the Shipwrecked Mariners Society.

The crew later returned to the stranded steamer to undertake repairs, and had to be rescued a second time by the rocket apparatus. The ship was left high and dry when the tide fell, and it was only after a considerable amount of sand and shingle had been bulldozed from around her that she was able to return to the sea.

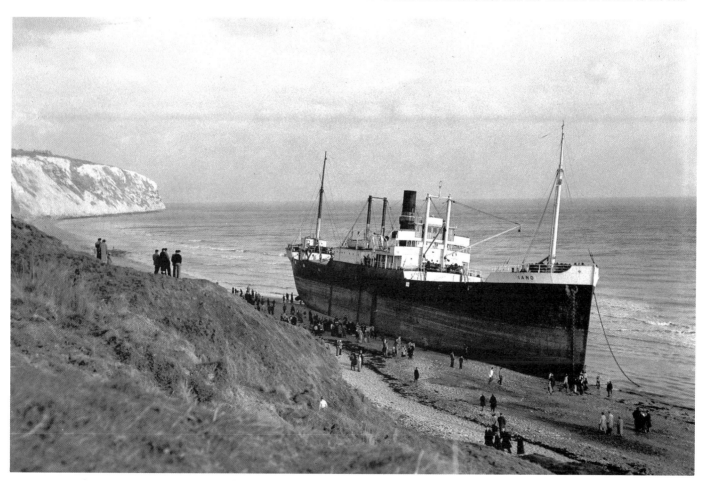

The stranded Iano. (Courtesy of Mrs. K. Wheeler).

Shipwrecks of the Sixties

The Brother George and the Witte Zee

The *Brother George* was one of the last big ships to come ashore on the Island's south-west coast. She was pulled off two days later, but in the process the Dutch tug *Witte Zee,* was holed and sank while struggling to reach the Needles Channel.

The *Brother George* was a 7,303 ton freighter, originally a 'liberty ship,' built in America in 1942 in a matter of weeks to bring supplies to Europe during the Battle of the Atlantic. On February 23rd, 1964, she was steaming in ballast from Manchester to her home port, Rotterdam, when she came ashore on Brook Ledge at 1.45 a.m. There was a heavy swell running but there was no danger to the crew who radioed for tugs.

At 8.45 that morning the new Yarmouth lifeboat the *Earl and Countess Howe* under acting coxswain Jim Simmonds, helped to pass a towing line from the Red Funnel tug *Gatcombe* to the stranded steamer, but the line slipped and the *Brother George* had to await the following tide.

As the day wore on, overcast and miserable with a heavy swell, two more tugs arrived, the *Abielle* from France and the *Witte Zee* of Messrs. Smit and Company, the oldest towing and salvage company in the world. As the *Witte Zee* came from Rotterdam, the steamer's home port, it was natural that they should get the salvage contract. The *Witte Zee* was a 327 ton

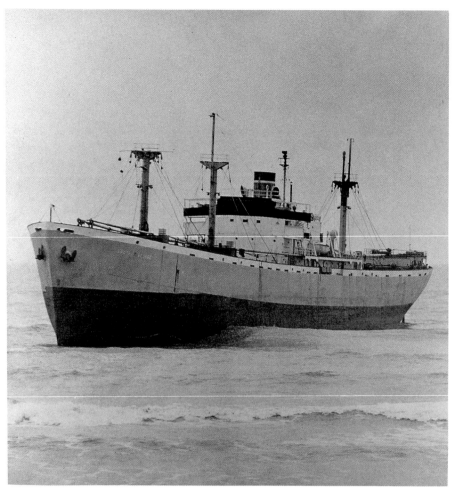

The Brother George, ashore at Brook.

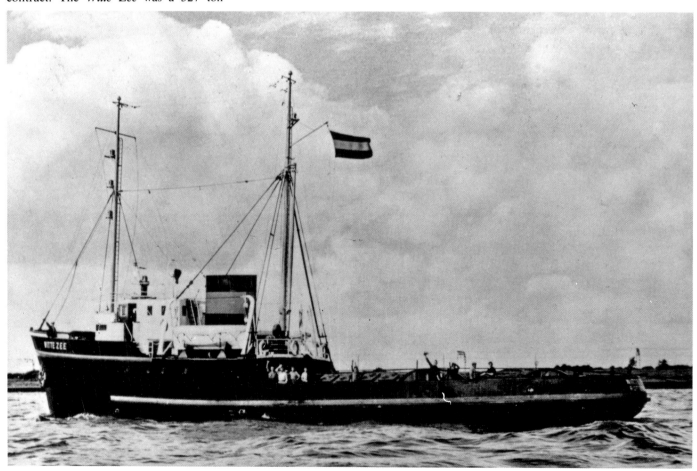

The Dutch tug Witte Zee, which was sunk while attempting to tow off the Brother George. (Courtesy of Gordon Phillips).

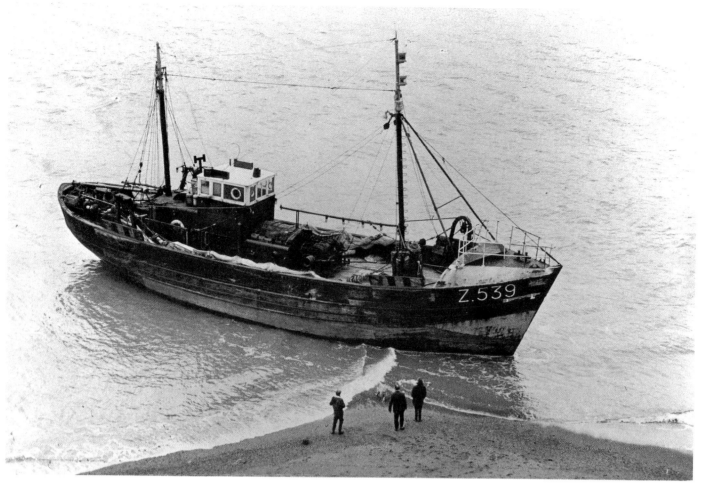

The Belgian trawler Zeemansblik close to the shore at Atherfield Point.

ocean going tug, just a year younger than the *Brother George*, with motors that could produce 1,000 horse power.

Her Master, Captain Kleyn, decided that he would fire a line to the steamer before the tide reached high water at 8 p.m. He carefully closed the *Witte Zee* towards the shore until she was close enough to fire. While the crew were engrossed in firing the rocket a particularly large swell came up behind the tug. Just as the rocket smoke-cloud cleared in the breeze, the wave struck the tug, breaking over her stern. "She rolled heavily to port under the blow, and instead of righting herself immediately there was an appreciable delay before she returned to an even keel." The tug was badly damaged, a hole punched in her bow and flooding her supposedly watertight hull. Kleyn swung his ship around and headed for the Needles, he knew his best chance lay in getting his crippled ship to the Solent and then beaching her. However, the water flooded in too quickly. Two miles off Compton the *Witte Zee* radioed for help.

Luckily for Kleyn and his crew the *Earl and Countess Howe* was heading straight towards them, on its way to watch over the salvage of the *Brother George*. The other tugs also came to Kleyn's assistance. Eight of the *Witte Zee's* crew were taken off by the *Gatcombe* and the *Abeille* took the crippled tug in tow. When the lifeboat came alongside the *Witte Zee* she was low in the water and hard to control. The two vessels crashed together in the swell, causing considerable damage to the lifeboat's starboard side. Kleyn was the last man to abandon his ship at 9 p.m., by then the tug's decks were awash. The men aboard the *Gatcombe* were transferred to the *Earl and Countess Howe* which then returned to Yarmouth. The *Witte Zee* finally foundered at 11 p.m. in a dense swirling mist, about four miles from Compton.

The following day two more Smit and Co. tugs arrived and the *Schelde* pulled off the *Brother George* that evening. The ship was not seriously damaged and was towed to Rotterdam for repairs.

The Zeemansblik

A year after the loss of the *Witte Zee*, the Belgian trawler *Zeemansblik* came ashore at Atherfield. She was just returning

from a 16 day fishing trip in the Bristol Channel, with seven tons of fish packed in ice, when she went ashore on the ledge at 10 p.m. on February 21st, 1965. It was a clear night but there was a heavy swell running and breaking over the trawler's stern. One big sea washed away her life-raft and Captain Vandierendonck radioed for help, calling out the L.S.A. crew and the Yarmouth lifeboat. Luckily for the five crew the life-raft was washed back to them by another sea and they were able to abandon their ship. They were picked up by a coastal tanker which had heard their distress call. Later they were transferred to the *Earl and Countess Howe* and safely brought to Yarmouth.

By the following morning the *Zeemansblik* had been pushed up to within 15 yards of the shore, and was embedded in sand in an upright position. She was badly damaged. The crew went home except for Vandierendonck who stayed on to sell the uninsured cargo. His battered vessel remained on the rocks where it was broken up by salvors.

Submarine Ashore

One unusual Island shipwreck which can be visited by the public is the 'A' Class submarine *Alliance*. During exercises in the Channel she went aground on Bembridge Ledge on January 13th, 1968. When the tide fell the submarine was left stranded high and dry on the ledge. The crew were taken off by helicopter and the *Alliance* was refloated the following day by two naval dockyard tugs and a salvage ship. The *Alliance* is now on display at the Gosport Submarine Museum.

The Modern R.N.L.I.

With the obvious decline in the number of serious wrecks it might be wondered if the two lifeboat stations at Yarmouth and Bembridge have any purpose. In fact they are busier than ever. Both have made repeated rescues from ships, yachts and dinghies in trouble in the Solent, or cliff climbers or swimmers taking too great a risk. Between 1938 and 1977 the Yarmouth Station rescued no less than 307 people, and from 1939 to 1970 the Bembridge Station saved another 289 people's lives.

Near Catastrophe: The Pacific Glory

The greatest environmental threat to the Isle of Wight was the wreck of the 43,000 ton Liberian super tanker *Pacific Glory*. On October 23rd, 1970, she suffered a collision and a series of explosions just three miles off the Island's southern coast, killing one third of the crew and causing a blazing inferno that nearly released 70,000 gallons of crude oil onto the Island's precious beaches. An ecological disaster was only averted by the most extensive sea rescue operation in the region's history.

The drama began at 9 p.m. on that Friday evening in October when the Hong Kong based super tanker was steaming up Channel towards Rotterdam with a cargo of 70,000 gallons of African crude and a crew of 42 under Captain Chan Shih Pian. At that time he had given over command to the recently boarded Dutch pilot, J. Frudiger. When the *Pacific Glory* was six miles off St. Catherine's the men on the bridge were stunned to see the 46,000 ton tanker *Allegro* veering towards them out of the dusk in an effort to avoid a collision with a third ship. These tankers are so vast that they take a mile to respond to the helm, and the crews of both ships could only watch the *Allegro's* huge bow plough into the *Pacific Glory's* starboard side, cutting a deep wound amidships. Frudiger ordered the engines to stop and the lifeboats to be made ready. The giant cripple drifted towards Ventnor on the incoming tide, her crew busy dealing with the vessel's injuries. The *Allegro* continued her journey to Fawley where she was later arrested pending investigations on the accident.

Terrific Explosion

During the collision fuel oil pipes leading to the *Pacific Glory's* engine room had been severed and at 10.30 the escaping fuel erupted into a terrific explosion. Second Officer Chupui Sang was below: "Suddenly the lights went out and the ship was shaking." The force of the explosion ripped through the tanker's decks in a 80 foot sheet of flame which lit the darkness for miles around. Four men and a boy standing on the poop were killed instantly and many of the crew were injured. Two more explosions followed and soon the great ship was engulfed in thick black smoke from a fire amidships. Oil spurted through a hole on the starboard side igniting on the water, and slowly surrounding the doomed ship with a

burning halo of death. Frudiger and the crew made no attempt to fight the fire, already eight men were dead and almost everyone injured. They abandoned ship immediately, most like Chupui Sang diving into the water and swimming out through the choking oil. Five more drowned or perished in the burning oil.

By 11 p.m. the floating inferno was just three miles off Ventnor, threatening to erupt into more explosions or split apart disgorging her main cargo, and thus ending the Island's tourist industry at a stroke. Luckily the bulkheads between the various holds held firm until the fire-fighting tugs arrived from Fawley to fight the blaze and cool the tanker's hull.

The response to the disaster was magnificent. From the Royal Navy's H.Q. at Portsmouth, 'Operation Solfire' swung into action. The combined services of the Navy, Portsmouth and Southampton Fire Brigades, the Coastguard, hospitals, R.N.L.I., Police, local councils and the R.S.P.C.A. were mobilised and co-ordinated to meet the challenge. While the fire fighting tugs fought the blaze on the sea, naval and salvage ships, the two Island lifeboats, helicopters and a military hovercraft surrounded the glowing inferno, lighting the scene with flares and searchlights and rescuing the 29 survivors from the polluted sea. They were all rushed to Haslar naval hospital suffering from broken bones, burns, shock and swallowed oil.

The struggle against the floating inferno continued throughout the night as it slowly retreated towards the open sea on the falling tide. For the moment the Island was saved. After an intense three hour struggle the firemen aboard the tugs doused the conflagration on the sea, and then brought the fire on board under control.

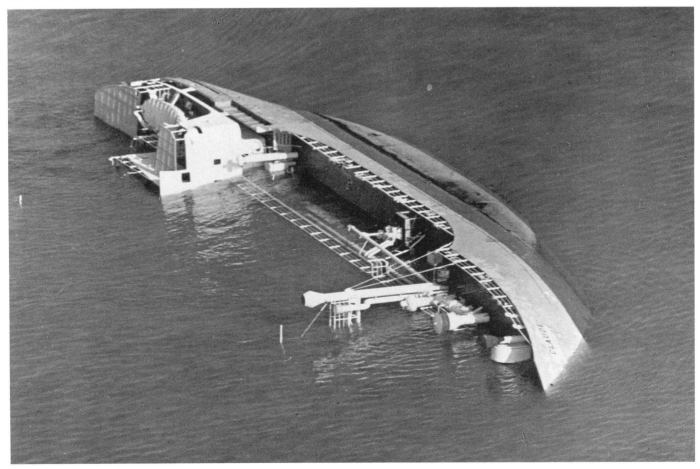

The 1,244 ton motor tanker Claude capsized on the Brambles after a collision with the M.V. Darlington off Yarmouth on September 25th, 1969.

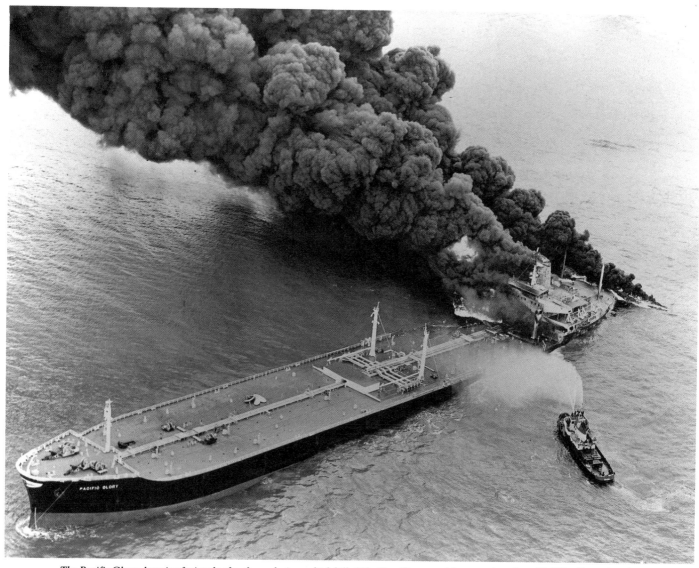

The Pacific Glory, burning furiously after the explosions which killed 13 of her 42 crew and threatened to release 70,000 gallons of crude oil onto the Island's beaches. (Courtesy of Portsmouth and Sunderland Newspapers).

The following morning the cripple was gently pushed towards Sandown Bay by a number of tugs. They hoped to ground her in the relatively sheltered shallows of Nab Shoal, off Bembridge. She was still buoyant at the bows, but her stern was well down in the water, her towering blackened superstructure being lapped by the sea; the aft decks awash.

All seemed well until the smouldering fire burst into new life. A thick pillar of black smoke rose into the sky; by midday it was several miles high. The tugs hurriedly dumped the wreck onto a sandbank one mile off Dunnose Point.

The battle against the fierce oil fire went on all day, the firemen had to stop the ship breaking up and releasing its horrific cargo into Sandown Bay. On the Island 500 men stood by with 8,000 gallons of special detergent while the coastguards and the R.S.P.C.A. patrolled the beaches. Thankfully none of the oil reached the Island, the threatening slicks being broken up by ships spraying detergent. The firemen's battle with the roaring furnace aboard the tanker continued throughout Saturday, on through the night and finally ended on Sunday afternoon. To the surprise and relief of everyone, the hull of the *Pacific Glory* remained intact.

The Ship That Would Not Die

Just when the tanker seemed safe a new danger arose. By the time that the fire was out the wind was rising to a force 8 gale, which generated a big swell that hammered the ship and the flotilla of ships fighting the fire and the oilslicks. The 70 ton *Beaulieu* nearly foundered with 40 reporters on board, only escaping thanks to *H.M.S. Zulu* intervening to mask her from the wind so that she could turn and escape. The tug *Harry Sharman* was less lucky, running straight into the base of Culver Cliff. Her Master refused a tow, arousing speculation that he was more interested in the insurance than saving the vessel. Within a few years the tug had almost completely disappeared.

Somehow the *Pacific Glory* stood up to this battering from the sea. When Rear Admiral Power told the press that the hull was still intact on Monday morning the reporters re-christened her 'the ship that wouldn't die.' That morning the final battle began as the Portsmouth Fire Brigade boarded the wreck having learned the detailed layout of the tanker's compartments and ventilation shafts from the ship's officers. They soon made sure that the fire was properly extinguished and then handed over to a Belgian and Dutch salvage team. From Thursday onwards the salvors were able to pump out the ship's main cargo into smaller tankers moored alongside, removing at last the fear of an ecological disaster of unimaginable consequences.

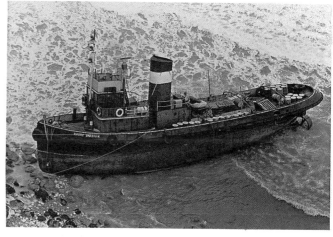

The tug Harry Sharman, grounded under Culver Cliff during the struggle against the Pacific Glory. She became a total wreck. (Courtesy of Portsmouth and Sunderland Newspapers).

Acknowledgements

This book in its present form was made possible through the help and generosity of the following Institutions and individuals.

Cowes Maritime Museum.
Carisbrooke Castle Museum.
The Royal National Lifeboat Institution.
The Department of Trade and Industry.
The Mary Rose Trust.
The Isle of Wight County Archaeological Centre.
The Isle of Wight County Records Office.
The City of London Guildhall Library.
The National Maritime Museum, Greenwich.
Beken of Cowes.
Gordon Phillips.
Geoffrey Cotton.
Mike Rayner.
Dave Wheeler.
Robin McInnes.

The Imperial War Museum, Lambeth.
H.M. Coastguards.
The Royal Naval Museum, Portsmouth.
The Admiralty Wreck Department, Taunton.
The Isle of Wight County Press.
Trinity House.
Portsmouth and Sunderland Newspapers.
Wright and Logan, Naval Photographers, Portsmouth.
The Needles Underwater Archaeology Group.
The International Ship Society.
Bembridge Maritime Museum.
Gordon Wheeler.
Tom Rayner.
Andy Butler.
Viv Spencer.

With particular thanks to the Blackgang Chine Museum which provided the photographs for pages, 5, 14, 20, 23, 26, 29, 32, 33, 34, 35, 38, 40, 43, 44, 45, 46, 47, 48, 49, 51, 63, 64, 66 and 67.

Bibliography

Back of the Wight	G. F. Mew B.E.M.
The Channel Shore	Aubrey de Selincourt
Waters of the Wight	Douglas Phillips-Birt
Solent Hazards	Peter Bruce
Insula Vecta	S. F. Hockey
The Mary Rose	Margaret Rule
The Story of the Mary Rose	Ernle Bradford
Isle of Wight Bedside Anthology	Hugh Noyes
The Dutch East Indiaman Campen	(Editor) Richard Larn
Island Longshoremen	Richard Hutchings
The Loss of the Royal George	Brigadier R. F. Johnson
Shipwreck at Goose Rock: The Discovery and Excavation of the Georgian frigate Pomone on the Needles of the Isle of Wight	Dr. D. Tomalin and P. Simpson (forthcoming publication)
The Journal of the Royal National Lifeboat Institution	
Dictionary of Disasters at Sea During the Age of Steam 1824-1962	(Editor) C. Hocking
Rowing Lifeboats of the Western Wight (Serialised in the Islander Magazine)	Geoffrey Cotton
The Book of Shipwrecks	Hudson and Nicholls
Stories of the Lifeboat	Frank Mundell
Launch	General Seely, later Lord Mottistone
Shipwrecks Around Britain	Leo Zanelli
Unknown Shipwrecks Around Britain	Leo Zanelli
British Vessels Lost at Sea 1914-1918	Pat Stevens
Fifty Years of Yarmouth, Isle of Wight Lifeboats	Geoffrey Cotton
British Vessels Lost at Sea 1939-1945	Pat Stevens
Board of Trade Wreck Inquiries	

Newspapers

Lloyds Lists
The Isle of Wight County Press
The Isle of Wight Guardian
The Evening Echo

The Illustrated London News
The Times
The Isle of Wight Mercury
The Portsmouth Evening News

Front Cover Illustration: "The Wreck of the Irex" by Felicity Joan Edwards
Back cover photograph: The tug Priscilla aground at Compton Bay